VEGETARIAN MEDICINES

OTHER BOOKS BY CLARENCE MEYER
Available from the Publisher

AMERICAN FOLK MEDICINE
50 YEARS OF THE HERBALIST ALMANAC
THE HERBALIST, Revised Edition
HERBAL RECIPES: For Hair, Salves &
Liniments, Medicinal Wines and Vinegars.

VEGETARIAN MEDICINES

Written & Compiled by
CLARENCE MEYER

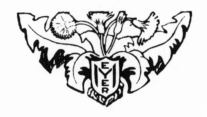

MEYERBOOKS
Glenwood, Illinois

Cover and plant illustrations were drawn by the author

Published by
Meyerbooks
P. O. Box 427
235 West Main Street
Glenwood, Illinois 60425

ISBN 0–916638–06–5

Second Printing

Table of Contents

v

Publisher's Note

Today the use of over-the-counter drugs has become the way of life for many people. Drugs are not permitted to be marketed unless approved, having definite potency for claims made. Long term use, over-use, or in chemical combinations sometimes may have marked influence upon health.

The aim of this book is to show how people in the Old World, in domestic and orthodox practice, have used and still use fruits and vegetables for assorted conditions. Many simple recipes may be used by the layman for minor conditions beneath the doctor's attention. Chronic ailments, diseases and special diets should be treated or supervised only by a physician.

Neither author nor publisher vouch for any claims made in this book.

Preface

Most of us have heard the old saying, "An apple a day keeps the doctor away." The doctor is not kept away merely by munching this fruit. The health properties of the apple depend largely on how it is used; the kind of apple eaten; its ripeness; how the raw fruit is chewed, cooked, brewed, or fermented. The apple is one of nature's most useful of all fruits. It can be used with benefit for many conditions—minor or serious—as well as a preventive measure or simply as a food to help maintain health. Apples, when properly prepared, usually can be tolerated from infancy to old age, in convalescence, debility or as a nonfattening and refreshing snack.

The earliest mention of the apple was in the Bible when Eve offered the forbidden fruit to Adam. Apples were on earth since remote antiquity but not used for their therapeutic potentials until recent times while the beneficial properties of other plant foods were recognized some 5,000 years or more ago. Garlic, onions, cabbage, radish, and spices were used as medicinals by all the ancient civilizations. Hippocrates, the most celebrated physician of antiquity, wrote: "Thy food shall by thy remedy." The renowned School of Salerno, earliest and oldest medical school in Christian Europe, considered plant foods equally as important for their therapeutic properties as plants used solely as medicinals.

In modern Europe food plants are still much used with plant medicines in spas, sanatoriums and in orthordox and folk practice. In city and town apothecaries one may find plant medicines used since ancient times on shelves with products of the chemical age. In grocery stores and outdoor markets medicinal plants are often offered with food plants. In rural gardens folk still grow necessary simples with their vegetables, fruits and flowers. Families use medical recipes handed down from one generation to another. Simple home recipes may often avert conditions that could lead to more serious ailments if not treated in the early stages. In areas far from professional help it is necessary to be prepared for emergencies or accidents in the house or farm. The excruciating pain of burns needs a palliative as soon as possible that cannot wait for professional help from distant places. Cuts, wounds, bruises, bee or wasp stings and other painful conditions need immediate attention. Common ailments such as constipation, diarrhea, colds, coughs, sore throat, nosebleed, aches and pains and ailments beneath the attention of doctors are often successfully treated in home practice. Several priests who made weekly or monthly rounds to tiny chapels tucked in remote valleys of Bavarian and Swiss Alps achieved a reputation for their successful treatments of ailing parishioners with food and plant medicines found at hand.

Many people living in crowded European cities still maintain an inseparable relationship with nature. If a bit of soil is wedged between buildings, dwellers plant flowers, vegetables, herbs or a small tree. Windowsills and balconies are often crowded with potted plants. In Munich, Germany, many folks maintain small garden plots on the outskirts of the city for their pleasure and relaxation as well as providing for the kitchen. On weekends and holidays there is a mass exodus from the city to parks, farms, woodlands, lakesides and mountains where people walk or hike to clear the lungs and enjoy the serenity only God and nature can provide. Nature's products and her environments are essential to man's life, health and mental well being.

PART I
Eighteen Common Food Plants & How They Have Been Used Medicinally

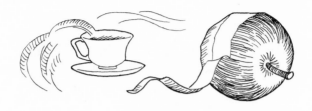

Apple

A well known health enthusiast, who has retained her beauty and wit with age, said the best apple was one with a worm in it. This, of course, implied that a worm would not eat an apple sprayed with deadly chemicals or coated with "eye appeal" substances. German and Austrian medical writers believe the best apples are the common varieties that have not been highly changed by the hybridizing of horticulturists. They contend that the green or yellow colored hybridized fruits, although pulpy and tasty, lack much of the beneficial qualities of the commoner types.

Alexander Nelson of the University of Edinburgh wrote that the important vitamin C content of "dessert varieties" of apples is generally poor; the "culinary varieties" have a rather high vitamin C content but the "cider varieties" have the highest content of vitamin C of all. It is quite obvious that much of the latter vitamin content is because cider apples must also be thoroughly ripe. The vitamins and minerals of apples are concentrated mainly near the peel. The rosey side exposed to the direct sun contains the most virtues. To obtain the qualities of the peel, it must be slowly and thoroughly chewed. In Europe apple peels are dehydrated and brewed to make a delicious and healthful tea.

People who cannot tolerate raw apples because of flatulence tendency (which they sometimes occasion), may find the fruit more agreeable by eating it with bread. Apples contain fruit acids, gallotannic acid, pectin, vitamins A, B, C, fruit sugars, minerals, trace elements and metabolism-promoting properties.

• • • • • • •

Dr. Fernie wrote: "Cider drinkers during epidemics of cholera have been found to singularly escape the disease. Cider being powerfully antiseptic because of its methyl-aldehyde content."

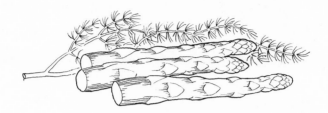

Asparagus

"This is considered to be one of the most wholesome, and at the same time agreeable products of the garden. It is strongly diuretic and at the same time sedative. The frequent use of it in its green state, as an article of food, has been strongly recommended, not only for persons who require diuretics but also in affections of the chest and lungs. It is used medicinally, when no longer in season, but preserving it in the same way as any other green vegetable, or drying it and reducing it to powder, or making an extract. The extract is made by boiling asparagus in water several hours, then straining the liquor and evaporating it slowly over a very low fire until it becomes exceedingly thick. Two or three tablespoonfuls of good brandy are then added to each quarter of a pint of this extract to preserve it and it is put by in bottles for use. A tablespoonful of it may be used night and morning, in water or milk," *The Domestic Dictionary* by G. Merle and J. Reitch, M.D., 1842. Asparagus contains saponin, asparagin, rutin, tannin, calcium and trace elements.

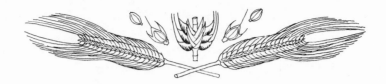

Barley

Long before wheat was cultivated, barley was the "staff of life" for all the ancient civilizations of the Old World. No less than three varieties were used by the prehistoric Lake Dwellers of Europe. Hippocrates, "Father of Medicine," recommended a daily drink of barley water and the prescription has retained its popularity after almost 2,000 years of use. *The Oxford Medical Adviser* by J. D. Comrie, physician and lecturer, gives the following recipe for barley water: "Simmer 2 ounces of pearl barley in a quart of water for 2 hours. Add enough sugar to sweeten and lemon juice to flavor, strain. Taken cold, the water is very soothing for sore throat. It is also used as a food instead of milk, and as a cooling drink in fevers and in kidney disorders." Barley seedlings are rich in vitamins B_1 and E. The grain contains 70 to 80 percent protein, fats, starch and enzyme. Barley sprouts contain the valuable alkaloid hordenin and aminophenol.

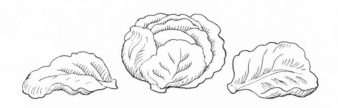

Cabbage, White

Cabbage was already an important crop in the time of Greek and Roman civilizations. The vegetable probably was brought to these countries by conquering Roman legions from northern Europe where the plant was cultivated for ages before by Germans, Saxons and Celts. Cabbage was a panacea in Cato's time as well as a cure-all for Germanic races. Despite the modern introduction of new foods and exotic drugs from the world over, the German esteem for their vegetable has not been diminished in the least. Cabbage and sauerkraut are their favorite foods and still regarded a cure-all by many rustics. The plant is mentioned in all old herbals for a variety of therapeutic conditions. Modern researchers are confirming some folk practices and also discovering new uses and potentialities. An early modern use was mentioned in W. Rhind's *A History of the Vegetable Kingdom* (1868). He wrote: "Sauerkraut has been found of sovereign efficacy as preservative from scurvy during long voyages. It was for many years used in our navy for this purpose, until displaced by lemon juice, which is equally a specific, while it is not so bulky an article for store." An American authority added in 1937 that cabbage is one of the best protective foods, for it contains the antiscorbutic vitamin and is also rich in sulfur.

A 1953 report states cabbage juice and the concentrates contain large amounts of an unidentified diet factor called vitamin U, which is believed to fortify the digestive tract against the onslaught of pepsin. Pepsin is a digestive enzyme contained in

7

the stomach juices that bore into tissues under certain conditions causing peptic ulcers.

In 1961 researchers reported a common amino acid found in cabbage juice has been used with good results in the treatment of alcoholism and peptic ulcers.

Findings of the University of Giessen (Germany) state that sauerkraut contains 1.5 percent lactic acid, which has direct action upon colon flora and spares the normal coli flora and suppresses the bacteria that cause illnesses. It also contains acetyhicholin, an agent for the normal action of the bowels. In European folk practice the calcium, iron, and vitamin-rich bruised outer leaves of white cabbage are much used externally as an application for skin diseases, burns, ulcers, boils, hemorrhoids, wounds, neuralgia, sciatica, lumbago, etc.

As a food, a veritable vegetable garden has been developed through the ages from the wild cabbage which is still found growing along the seacoasts of England. Through selection, mutation or hybridization we have white and red cabbages. Near Regensburg, Germany, the author saw a robust purplish blue variety of cabbage growing in a garden. Savoy cabbage, chinese cabbage, kahls, Brussel sprouts, broccoli, kohlrabi and cauliflower are all related to the seacoast weed. In recent years a beautiful flower-like cabbage used as an ornamental was developed by the Japanese.

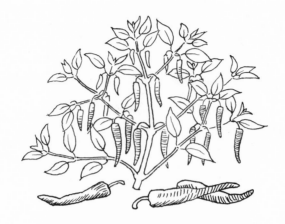

Cayenne Pepper

The fiery pungency of this pepper is never forgotten when once tasted in its natural form. Cayenne peppers are derived from the pulverized ripe fruits of *Capsicum fastigiatum, C. frutescens* and *C. minimum*. The hot-flavored fruits are related to sweet peppers, paprikas, bell peppers and numerous other species commonly used as food or condiment, especially in the tropics.

Cayenne pepper is a highly regarded medicinal in domestic and orthodox practice. The powdered fruit or extract is used in liniments, ointments and plasters as a counter-irritant against chilblains, rheumatism and neuralgia. Cayenne pepper taken internally in moderate doses as a stimulant produces a pleasant feeling of warmth and is often preferable to alcoholic stimulants such as brandy and whiskey. The spice is also beneficial as a carminative in flatulence and dyspepsia.

"Cayenne pepper made into pills with bread has been used in indigestion with excellent results, but it is a remedy not to be trifled with. Generally speaking, however, the patient is the best judge as to whether it should be continued. If he does not find any immediate and unpleasant effects from its use, he may increase the dose to any extent, according to his sensations. Cayenne pepper is not one of those things which gives direct evidence of its action; it either does good immediately, or harm, and must be abandoned, or preserved in according to the indications which the patient receives. Cayenne pepper is used much more extensively in warm than cold countries, and seems there to be essential to keep up the equilibrium of heat between the surface and the interior of the body. The quantity of pepper used in some warm climates would be injurious in the colder parts of Europe," *The Domestic Dictionary* by G. Merle and J. Reitch, M.D., 1842.

Cayenne pepper is also known as red pepper and capsicum. It is used in curries, hot pepper sauces, stews, pickles, etc.

Cayenne pepper contains capsaicin (vanillylamid of methylnonen acid), volatile oil, vitamins A, C, and citrin.

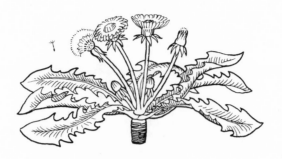

Dandelion

Dandelion is one of the most valuable nutritional plants of the northern hemisphere and is particularly esteemed by all races living along the northern slopes of the Alps. Early colonists brought this plant to the New World where it is now considered a nuisance and treated with herbicides. Recently botanists have removed dandelion's *T. officinale* (recognized medicinal) title and dubbed it *Taraxacum vulgare.* In European orthodox and folk practice the therapeutic properties are still held in high esteem.

Dandelion leaves are rich in vitamins B complex, C, and exceptionally rich in vitamin A (more than carrots). The leaves contain folic acid and protein in amounts comparable to spinach. The greens are an excellent source of iron, calcium, potassium and chlorophyll. The fresh leaves are much used as a blood purifier and in "Frühlingskur" (*See Spring Cure*). Dandelion roots contain inulin, resin, mucilage and the bitter principle taraxacin, and taraxacerin. The roots are regarded as one of the best known cholagogues (bile promoting agents). They are also used as a tonic, simple bitter, diuretic, and aperient, especially in dyspepsia arising from a torpid liver.

11

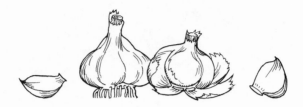

Garlic

The fact that garlic is grown over most of the world indicates its value not only as a condiment but also for its wide use as a medicinal. Garlic is generally not prescribed by the profession in the form the world's greatest Chemist made it. The entire garlic plant has a strong, rich and penetrating odor. It contains a volatile oil with allicine, diallylsulfide and other sulfides, alliinase enzyme, various ferments, and vitamins A, B_1, and B_2 nicotinamide complex. Garlic is a stomachic, antispasmodic and carminative. It has an antiseptic action on the stomach, a prophylactic action against amebic dysentery, typhus and other infectious diseases. Garlic has a favorable action on high blood pressure and is widely used to help prevent arteriosclerosis. Since ancient times garlic has been used as a medicinal for a variety of ailments, particularly in folk practice.

•   •   •   •   •   •   •

A German recipe book states people who eat raw garlic have strong clear voices. This may be the reason why the majority of the world's greatest singers were Italians who loved this condiment.

•   •   •   •   •   •   •

Garlic sniffed into the nostrils will revive an hysterical sufferer—a whiff puts some people to flight.

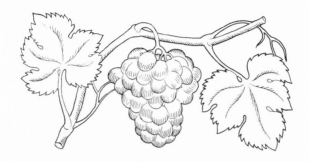

Grapes

In a 1977 report, two Canadian microbiologists found that grapes, grape juice, raisins and wines show anti-viral activity in the test tube. Strawberries and other fruits also contain various natural compounds with anti-viral activity. The researchers said the anti-bacterial properties of wine have been attributed to natural chemicals found in grapes, such as tannic acid and phenols. Since ancient times grapes and wines have been used for their healing properties. Roman soldiers washed wounds with wine and Egyptian warriors mixed wine with unfamiliar waters of countries they invaded.

• • • • • • •

Another report states that at the University of Stockholm, Von Euler, Nobel prize winner in chemistry, found that juices of lemons, black currants and other fruits contain a substance which is effective in preventing infection of pneumonia.

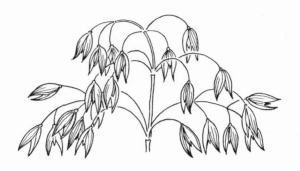

Oats

Oats contain more calcium and various other mineral sub-. stances than all other cereals. The grain contains 55 percent starch, 2 to 5 percent sugar, 10 percent protein and 5 percent fat. The grain also contains vanillosid, a substance that has an effect upon the central nervous system. Besides being used as a strengthening diet in debility and for diabetics, oats are used against dyspepsia and gastroenteritis. Anshutz wrote: "Oats is one of the most valuable means for overcoming the effects of morphine habit. Also: Oats appear to have a special sphere of action upon male sexual organs, regulating the functional irregularities of these parts perhaps as much as any drug can." Konrad Kölbl, a German writer, also believed oats beneficial for impotence.

• • • • • • •

Researchers at the University of Wisconsin discovered oats help cure the ulcers of a high-strung pig, but corn made it worse. Food rations containing 85 percent oats seem to prevent ulcers, but rations containing a substantial amount of corn caused a high incidence of stomach abnormalities in pigs. Pigs have long been known to develop ulcers from the stress of living in close quarters on modern farms.

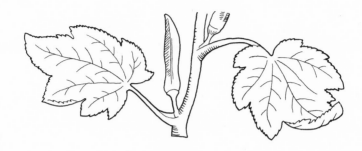

Okra

A 1952 News Item: "Like humans, animals frequently need blood plasma after severe shock. A substitute has been proven very successful in the laboratory. An extract from the okra pod is inexpensive, easily purified and may be stored indefinitely. It would have great value following operations, prolonged illnesses or accidents in animals. The okra extract is also being studied as a blood plasma substitute for humans." Since the news item appeared no further reports have been available.

· · · · · · ·

An East Indian physician that wrote okra forms an ideal vegetable food for the weak and the invalid and for those suffering from neurasthenia, beriberi and sleeplessness.

· · · · · · ·

Okra is much used in New Orleans and environs in creole and cajun dishes such as chicken and seafood gumbo soups. Okra is valued in the diet chiefly because of nutritionally important minerals. It is a good source of calcium, phosphorus and a fair source of iron. Fresh green okra is also a good source of vitamin A; however, drying reduces this content to about half.

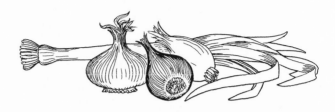

Onions

The following interesting excerpt was taken from Dr. W. T. Fernie's *Meals Medicinal:* "The onion has a very sensitive organism, and serves to absorb all morbid matter that comes in its way. It has been found that during an epidemic of cholera, a string of onions hanging in a house amid other houses which were all infected, became unintelligibly diseased, and black, but proving thereby protective to the inmates of that particular house." Culpepper tells about onions: "They have gotten this quality, to draw corruption unto them, for, if you peel one, and lay it on a dung hill, you shall finde him rotten in half a day by drawing putrefaction to it; then being bruised, and applied to a plague sore it is very probable it will do the like." The volatile principle of the bulbs, which is sulphide of allyl, is powerfully antiseptic whilst they are raw, but when boiled they lose their odorous essential oil in a great measure, on which the anti-putrefying virtues depend, and which escape by the heat. Onions also contain enzymes and vitamins A, B, and C, which are also partially or completely dissipated or destroyed by heat. The fresh juice of onions is bacteriostatic and choleric, it stimulates digestive juices and lowers blood pressure. In domestic practice the cooked onion is used against bladder complaints, colic, digestive troubles, hoarseness and inflamed throat. Recipe: Chop a medium-sized onion and cook it in a cup of water under low fire until it makes a thick juice. Strain and take a tablespoonful at a time.

. . . .

An old household medical guide says a Spanish onion fried in lard and applied locally makes a splendid poultice. Roasted in coals it makes a good poultice for earache, toothache, sore throat and sore chest.

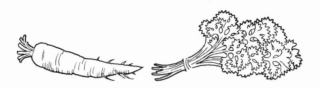

Parsley

The head of a European Institute of Nutrition wrote: "One can say without exaggeration that parsley is one of the most valuable nutritional products nature has given us." Professor Leon Binet considered the properties of parsley as extraordinary and believed its constituents to be an indisputable factor in maintaining youth and living a long life.

Parsley has been known since ancient times and was mentioned in the works of Dioscurides and Pliny The Elder.

The entire parsley plant, especially the seeds, contain a volatile oil with apiol and myristicin as the principle constituent. It also contains flavone, apiin, pinen, vitamin C, provitamin A and is exceptionally rich in minerals and trace elements. The root is diuretic, stomachic, emmenagogue and said to be an aphrodisiac. The decoction of the root or seed or the infusion of the leaves have been used in dropsy, yellow jaundice, coughing, asthma, amenorrhea and dysmeneorrhea.

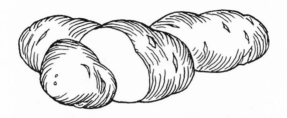

Potato

The entire potato contains the toxic alkaloid solanine but little in the starch of the tuber. The greatest accumulation of solanine is in the cells next to the skin, especially in the area which is green, and also the sprouts. Raw mature potatoes contain about 3 percent tannin, vitamins C, B_1, B_2, B_6 nicotinamide, pantothenic acid, organic acid acetylcholine and solanine starch. Much of the vitamins in potatoes are lost in cooking. The infinitesimal amount of solanine in potato starch after cooking is said to be entirely harmless. Raw potatoes, the water in which they are boiled and the steam are used in folk practices. *See Asthma, Skin and Wounds in Part II.*

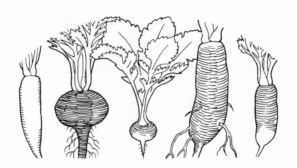

Radishes

Radishes were grown in Egypt more than 2,000 years ago and various forms are cultivated in most parts of the world. The red root variety is most highly esteemed and generally eaten raw for its pungent flavor. The black radish (also called the winter radish) is most prized by the Russians and the Germans as a food and medicinal. The root of this variety is larger than the common red types found in our markets. The root has a blackish skin and is firm fleshed. It is called winter radish as it can be stored for winter use.

Black radishes contain raphanin, an antibiotic anthocyanin, sulphur compounds, vitamins B_1, C, E and minerals. In European practice black radish is esteemed as a promoter of normal liver and gall bladder activity.

A 1957 News Item mentioned black radish pills being used in Europe to treat gall stones.

• • • • • •

Folk recipe for ailment of spleen: Take dessert-spoonful 3 or 4 times daily radish juice mixed with honey.

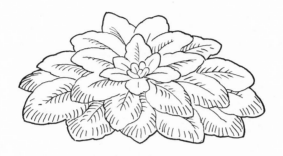

Spinach

The Oxford Book of Food Plants reported spinach is much richer in protein than other leaf vegetables. The leaves are also a superior source of minerals and an exceptional source of vitamins C, K_1, provitamin A, folic acid and chlorophyll. Spinach is an important addition in many diets for the sick and for infants and children. The folic acid of this leaf vegetable is said to have a counter effect against anemia. For vitamin deficiencies spinach is most useful eaten raw or drinking the juice. As a source of minerals the leaves may be boiled. Spinach is not recommended where there is rheumatism, arthritis, kidney stones and liver disease because of its high potassium and calcium oxalate content.

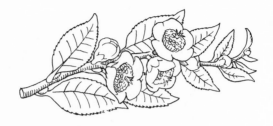

Tea

It was set forth in an ancient Chinese treatise on Materia Medica that tea "clears the voice, gives brilliancy to the eye, invigorates the constitution, improves the mental faculties, opens up the avenues of the body, promotes digestion, removes flatulence, and regulates the body temperature." Lin Yutang, noted modern author, believed tea prolongs Chinese lives by aiding their digestion and maintaining their equanimity of temper.

Tea has become the world's most popular beverage for "cups that cheer but not inebriate." Tea is often prescribed by modern physicians in medical diet and also used for a variety of conditions in domestic practice. The tea, as usually prepared, has stimulating and diuretic properties. Because of its low calorific value it is an excellent beverage for stout people, especially during the summer months to replace lost fluid from the body without adding fat to the tissues. The decoction (long boiling) of tea releases the strong tannin principle which makes an astringent gargle for relaxed mucous membranes. The decoction is taken internally to check diarrhea. The brew or moistened leaves are said to afford immediate relief for burns. Tea leaves are also used as a styptic for bleeding wounds and abrasions. Besides considerable tannin, tea contains from 1 to 5 percent caffeine, a trace of theophylline and boheic acid.

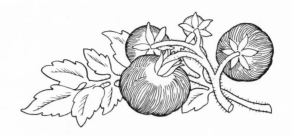

Tomato

Tomatoes were first known as love apples, golden apples or Peruvian apples. The plant is native to Central and South America and still found wild in that area. Tomatoes were brought to Spain by explorers in the 16th century and grown only as a novelty as they were believed to be poisonous. The luscious fruit probably tempted children as well as adults and when proved harmless, the use spread rapidly over Europe and eventually over much of the world.

As a medicinal, unsalted fresh vine-ripened tomatoes are believed helpful in the elimination of uric acid when eaten raw. The fruit had a long reputation of being beneficial to the liver, a corrective of biliary disorders, and an anti-scourbutic. Rustics used the ripe fresh tomato as a poultice for cleansing foul sores and to hasten maturation of gatherings or boils. The poultice was applied as hot as can be tolerated and renewed with fresh tomato after cooling.

Certain constituents in tomatoes appear to have deodorizing or cleansing properties according to a recent news item. The report stated that a cat encountered a skunk and returned home smelling to the high heaven. An ordinary bath was ineffective. Neighbors suggested using a folklore recipe which proved successful. The recipe: Bathe the animal with tomato juice, then follow with another bath of clear water to remove the tomato juice.

The entire tomato plant contains the alkaloid solanine but little in the ripe fruit. The fruit flesh contains the glucoside saponin, and the color matter lycopin and carotene, important amount of vitamin C, malic acid, several organic acids, fatty oil and histamine. Ripe tomato fruit contains about 94 percent water, therefore it is not nourishing; however, it is an excellent protective food when eaten raw because of its vitamin and mineral constituents. Many people are allergic to tomatoes because of its solanine, saponin and histamine content. The juice of the leaves and stems of tomatoes yield the antibiotic tomatin.

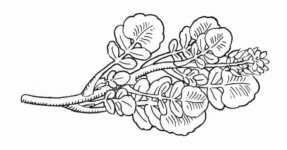

Watercress

Although the ancients did not know vitamins and minerals or other constituents of plants, they certainly did know the varieties most beneficial for the maintenance of health. Zenophon advised Persian mothers to feed their children watercress that they may grow tall and strong. "Eat more watercress and learn more wit" was a popular proverb of Greek and Roman times. Gerarde wrote in 1536: "Water Cresse being boiled in wine or milke, and drunk for certaine daies togither, is very good against the scurvie or scorbute." He also recommended watercress being boiled in meat broth to cure young maidens of the greensickness. The 1884 edition of *The National Dispensatory* states: "Watercress is still used in the spring to eliminate the crude humors accumulated during the winter. It increases the appetite, renders the bowels freer, and the urine more abundant."

This writer noted that watercress was grown in considerable quantities in Trinidad West Indies, apparently to help offset anemia commonly found among East Indian vegetarians.

An authoritative Austrian physician wrote that the liberal use of watercress in the diet helps prevent goiter and guards against infectious diseases. Goiter is prevalent in alpine regions of Europe.

Watercress contains glyconasturtiin, iodine, a bitter, vitamins C and E, minerals and trace elements. Medicinally the plant is regarded as a stimulant, diuretic and pectoral. It is widely used in folk practice as a stomachic, for bronchitis, skin troubles, poultices, loss of hair, etc.

Watercress should always be used in the fresh or raw state, as much of its active principles are lost in cooking.

PART II
Ailments & Conditions

ALCOHOLISM & INTOXICATION

Modern researchers found honey a cure for hangover as well as beneficial for acute intoxication. Honey contains a large amount of fructose, which promotes the chemical breakdown of alcohol. A Danish authority on alcoholism advised taking 4 ounces of honey slowly in a period of about 5 minutes. Take the same dose ½ hour later.

An old English doctor claimed a dish of stewed apples eaten 3 times daily worked wonders in cases of confirmed drunkenness and eventually gave the person an absolute distaste for alcohol in whatever form.

Dr. W. T. Fernie, author of *Meals Medicinal* (1905), wrote: "Very remarkable success attends the use of Cayenne pepper as a substitute for alcohol with hard drinkers, and as a valuable drug in *delirium tremens* when full doses given repeatedly at such intervals as seem necessary will reduce the tremor, and agitation within a few hours, causing presently a calm, prolonged sleep; at the same time the skin will become warm, and will perspire naturally; the pulse will subside in quickness, whilst regaining fullness, and volume; the kidneys also, and the bowels will act freely. For an intemperate person who really desires to wean himself from indulging in spirituous liquors, and yet feels to need some other stimulant in place thereof, at first Cayenne pepper, given in essence, or tincture, mixed with that of bitter orange peel, will answer most effectually, the doses being reduced in strength, and frequency from day to day. But no alcoholic liquor of any sort should be resumed; indeed, there will arise a mortal repugnance thereto . . . . For an attack of *delirium tremens*, beef tea redhot with Cayenne

29

pepper, and with grated Parmesan cheese in it, may be helpfully taken by the patient in frequent copious draughts. While this is so strong, and burning, that under ordinary conditions one would scarcely dare to taste it, yet the patient will pronounce it the most cool and refreshing drink."

Cayenne pepper is reputed to be the purest and most certain stimulant in herbal materia medica. It is also much used as a carminative, tonic and as a rubefacient. *See Cayenne Pepper in Part I.*

Some imbibers believe drinking milk absorbs and neutralizes the effects of alcohol. Another source advises sprinkling nutmeg on ice cold milk and drink slowly.

To get rid of excessive alcohol, drink warm water with salt to cause vomiting. This recipe is only effective if taken immediately after debauchery as alcohol is quickly absorbed into the system.

A 1972 news item from England: "Doctors at Middelsex Hospital have been investigating how to avoid that morning after feeling. Their conclusions: Stick to clear alcohols such as gin, white rum or vodka in preference to red wine, brown rum and whiskey, which are heavier in hangover-inducing elements."

Red currant juice in water enough to flavor is taken regularly as an "Ersatz" substitute for alcohol in Austria and Germany. The beverage is also much used by laborers doing heavy work to quench thirst. Red currant fruits contain hexoses, citric and malic acids, pectin, invertin and considerable amounts of vitamin C.

A family recipe book printed in 1822 offered the following: "The infusion made with cloves may be advantageously given in dyspepsia, particularly when it arises from the abuse of ardent spirits." Another spice recipe: Dyspeptic patients (from hard drinking) have been known to receive considerable benefit by drinking 1 or 2 cups of ginger tea for breakfast.

In India the liquid in which dates have been boiled is used to relieve intoxication.

Russians drink the juice of salted cucumbers after vodka imbibition.

Taken from a German spice book: "In Hungary a devilish sharp paprika schnapps is prepared and used not only for imagined or real ailments, but also claimed to help prevent drunkeness." Probably meaning no one would want to imbibe in this particular "bottled firewater."

Ancient Greeks and Romans also had recipes for heavy drinkers. Aristotle counseled his readers to "dine well on cabbage just before starting out for a big evening." Cato evidently preferred a form of cole slaw. He advised, "If you wish to drink much at a banquet, before dinner dip cabbage in vinegar and eat as much as you wish. When you have dined, eat 5 leaves. The cabbage will make you as fit as if you had had nothing, and you can drink as much as you will."

A French source states the juice of white cabbage is used for liver damaged by alcoholism.

Recipe from Charlemagne's time to prevent drunkenness: Saturate yourself first with garlic, then with your wine. The odorous recipe may not work on some modern wines that contain chemicals to reduce excess natural acids; chemicals to sterilize and preserve; chemicals to inhibit mold and secondary fermentation, etc.

APPETITE, Loss of
Bilberry juice with equal quantity of red wine and a little sugar makes a fine aperitif.

Another excellent aperitif is made with a small quantity of dried orange peels (not dyed) steeped for a week in red wine and sweetened to taste.

An aperitif rich in minerals and vitamins: Steep dried parsley herb in white wine for a week or more.

In small doses paprika stimulates the appetite and digestive juices.

A nibble of fresh watercress stimulates appetite.

Green onions also stir appetite.

APPLE DIET

Many health minded people in Europe follow an apple diet once a month to help keep the intestinal tract in a healthy condition. Recipes generally follow this regimen: For breakfast drink a glass of pure (no preservatives) apple juice mixed with juice of ½ lemon. Juices should not be chilled. Before lunch eat 1 or 2 apples with peel. At lunch drink the warm infusion of dried apple peel made like ordinary tea, sweetened with honey. Later eat 3 more apples with peels. At 4 or 5 o'clock drink more apple juice and in the evening eat a dish of applesauce sweetened with honey. The diet is taken also for gout, rheumatism, liver and kidney conditions, hardening of the arteries and early symptoms of old age. The pectin and pulp-cellulose constituents of apples have been described as acting somewhat like a sponge in the intestinal tract, absorbing decomposed wastes of metabolism and harmful micro-organisms and flushing them from the body. *See Apples in Part I.*

ARTERIOSCLEROSIS

The Grape Diet mentioned in this book was believed by Europeans to help hinder abnormal thickening and hardening of the arteries, providing the grape diet was followed in the early stages and the avoidance of alcohol, smoking and foods containing highly saturated oils was maintained.

In the Orient garlic is consumed with daily bread and is said to contribute much to the health of the people. Arteriosclerosis and high blood pressure are little known diseases. The meager consumption of meats, fats and certain other foods may also be important factors favorable in the Oriental diet.

Folk belief: Drink daily apple cider that has been boiled with garlic.

An authoritative German source reported the Russians eat mature raw potatoes at every meal as a precaution against arteriosclerosis. *See Potato in Part I.*

Paprika, also known as sweet pepper, is an important crop in Hungary and used in many native dishes. Hungarian researchers found there is less thickening and hardening of the arteries among rural folk who regularly eat considerable amounts of paprika in their diet. Paprika eaters are also reputed to live longer. People unaccustomed to paprika should not try to eat the condiment like the Hungarians. It may, however, be a health-contributing factor to use paprika in the salt-cellar instead of salt.

According to a French doctor, arteriosclerosis and cardiovascular diseases seldom occur among people who eat rye bread made with baker's yeast.

ASTHMA

People who eat an abundance of garlic or sauerkraut generally are least likely to have asthma, according to German sources.

In Russia the steam from boiling potatoes is inhaled for asthma.

A German doctor's recipe: Make a decoction by boiling parsley root and herb (tablespoonful of each) in a pint of water for 5 minutes. When lukewarm strain and drink 1 cupful.

In the evening, before retiring, take 1 teaspoon of minced fresh horseradish root with an equal part of honey. Another: Take 4 ounces of fresh horseradish root, add the juice of 1 fresh lemon.

Avoid mucus-forming foods such as dairy products, concentrated starchy foods, breads and cereals. Also avoid salt.

BITES & STINGS

Powdered mustard seed mixed with wine vinegar is an emergency application for animal and snake bites where doctors are not immediately available.

The bites of insects, dog or snakes are relieved by applying garlic juice to the wound, according to an Austrian source.

All poisonous bites should be treated by a physician as quickly as possible.

Grated or sliced fresh horseradish root quickly relieves the pain of bee, wasp or other insect bites. Bees leave a stinger in the skin—this must be removed before horseradish is applied.

The pain of bites from bees or wasps is quickly relieved by applying a slice of onion, potato, mashed cabbage leaf or wet salt.

In France the fresh blades of leeks, slightly mashed, are applied to insect bites and claimed to quickly relieve pain.

Apply honey to stings of bees after removing stinger.

Stings from jelly-fish, Portuguese man-of-war, or hairy caterpillars may be relieved by applying olive oil.

Unrefined barley meal heated with a little wine is used as a plaster for insect bites by peasants of the Old World.

Rub uncovered parts of the skin with fresh parsley as protection against insect bites. Another source states that the juice of parsley leaves is rubbed on mosquito and gnat bites.

BLOOD

Is the Fountain of Youth in a sauerkraut barrel? Konrad Kölbl believed raw sauerkraut not only purifies the blood but rejuvenates and lengthens life. Sauerkraut is rich in mineral elements especially basic in nature for the elimination of metabolic waste matters and for the utilization of nourishment. Kölbl recommended 2 dessert-spoonfuls of raw kraut on a little whole wheat bread.

Dr. A. F. M. Willich wrote in 1802: "Though modern physicians smile at the idea of buttermilk sweetening or purifying the blood, yet the good effects of buttermilk, as well as sweet whey, in proper cases and constituents, to admit any doubt, in consequences of an unsettled theory."

In Europe spinach is often recommended in the diet of people with blood disturbances. The leaves contain iodine, iron, chlorophyll and flavones, and are rich in calcium, vitamins C and K_1 and folic acid, which has an effect against anemia. Spinach vitamin A content is almost on a par with that of carrots.

Herbalists considered ripe (when skin turns yellow) cucumbers a blood builder and purifier. An old physician wrote, "If they were one degree colder, they would be poison." The doctor probably referred to green cucumbers so often used in salads and to make pickles. Cucumbers are especially rich in potassium and phosphorus.

Grape juice is an excellent source of iron and is effective in building up the hemoglobin in blood. Ten ounces of juice taken daily is said to prevent secondary anemia.

Carrot juice is esteemed as a blood purifier in Europe. Carrots contain glucose, sucrose and pectin and are rich in vitamins B_1, B_2, C, and provitamin A (carotene). Carrots also are a good source for calcium, phosphorus and potassium.

In folk practice a tablespoonful of raisins taken an hour before lunch and again before evening meal is believed to be beneficial for plethora.

Liberal use of garlic alone and in many foods is believed in European folk practice to thin and purify the blood as well as to be an effective preventative against many ailments. In Germany children are often given daily a few drops of garlic juice in their milk. Small amounts of garlic juice are also added to butter. Adults use wine and brandy in which several cloves of garlic have been steeped.

Garlic tablets are widely used to lower high blood pressure. The tablets are sold in Health Food Stores.

The juice or fruit of blackberries and strawberries have an old reputation for being blood purifying.

Fresh watercress eaten daily helps purify the blood. The herb is also popular as a "Frühlingskur." *See Spring Cure.*

Daily use of apples in the diet is believed to help keep the blood in healthy condition.

Chervil is esteemed as a blood purifier in France. The fresh chopped leaves are served in a saucer and sprinkled on salads, sauces, meats, stews, soups, sandwiches, and to garnish dishes. The leaves have a delicate anise-like flavor. The plant is easily grown and winter-hardy in the author's midwest garden. *See Spring Cure.*

The fresh pulp of pumpkin or squash is used in salads in Europe and reputed to have blood purifying properties. The cooked fruit loses this claimed property.

Excellent food sources for iron deficiency: Plums, raisins, garlic, chives, onions, leeks, strawberries, spinach, asparagus, kohlrabi, cabbage, radish, dandelion greens and watercress.

BOILS

In home practice thin slices of fresh pumpkin are applied to boils and abcesses to hasten suppuration. The application is changed frequently until the boil comes to a head.

The fresh green blades of leeks finely chopped added to a little milk or unsalted lard is used as a poultice for boils by Italian and French peasants. The application is heated and applied as hot as can be tolerated and renewed frequently with fresh leeks. The poultice is also used on carbuncles, and paronychia.

Cooked minced garlic applied as a poultice on a boil will remove the pus, according to Künzle. He also wrote that if one avoids meats and sour foods, boils as well as wounds will heal faster.

BRONCHIAL

An old Austrian recipe for bronchial catarrh and coughing: Fry finely cut onions in lard and apply to the chest at night.

The French make a cough syrup for bronchial catarrh by cooking equal weight of fresh blackberry juice with sugar. It is taken in tablespoonful doses as needed.

Russian recipe for bronchial catarrh: To 1 part black radish juice of root add 2 parts honey. Take a tablespoonful as needed. *See Radish in Part I.*

A German recipe: Take 5 to 10 drops of extract of garlic 3 times daily in water or vegetable juice. *See garlic extract recipe under heading FLU.*

Irish recipe: For chronic conditions use ½ oz. of carrageen (Irish moss), to 1½ pts. of water and boil down to 1 pt. This may be flavored with lemon or fruit juices. Carrageen is a popular food along coastal areas of Ireland. The refined product is now much used as a thickening agent for ice cream, chocolate milk, a homogenizer in dairy products, etc.

BURNS
Home remedies for the relief of pain from minor burns: Apply the leaves of white cabbage that have been softened by mashing lightly; apply sliced or minced onions to the part; dab burn with honey; a slice of raw potato (without peel), or the pulp of fresh pumpkin are cooling applications.

Minced clean fresh carrots applied to burns hastens the formation of scar tissue.

CHILDREN & INFANTS
This writer lived in Germany and has traveled through much of that country. The children appeared exceptionally healthy and strong. Pea soup is much used in German meals and may be a contributing health factor. The soup is especially fed to weak children and believed good for growth and bone building. Pea soup also is recommended for adults and especially for women in childbed.

Rolled oats cooked with 1 part water to 1 part milk makes a very good nourishing meal for growth, health and quiet sleep for children. Sweeten with honey.

From *Unsere Heil und Teepflanzen II:* Carrots are an indispensable home made remedy for children and baby's care.

Dr. Braun wrote that carrots are used in therapeutic practice for children and digestive disturbances of babies.

Olive oil taken in small doses like castor oil is a mild laxative for children.

Colic: Give baby in teaspoonful doses a warm infusion made with dill or fennel seeds. Steep a teaspoonful of either seeds in a cupful of boiling water. Strain when warm. Infusion may be sweetened.

A German folk recipe for wetting children: Give nothing to drink at bed-time; feet are placed higher than the head; apply brandy over abdominal area.

Black currant jelly in teaspoonful doses is useful for a child when suffering from thrush and sore throat.

From a home recipe book: For convulsive cough of children, spray pillow with wine vinegar.

Swiss home recipe for painful teeth: Bandage sliced onions to soles of feet.

Infant diaper rash: Apply honey to the baby's bottom.

A doctor's report on diarrhea in infants: Babies given carob flour in water every 4 hours were cured in about one-third the time it took babies being treated for diarrhea but not getting the carob flour. Another source mentions using boiling milk with carob flour instead of water. Boiled milk alone is often used for diarrhea. Carob, the fruit of a tree, is also called St. John's bread because it is believed the pods sustained John the Baptist in the desert. Carob flour needs no sweetening as it contains from 40 to 50 percent sugar. The pods also contain 6 percent protein, vitamin B and minerals. The pods are often available in city fruit markets and the flour at Health Food Stores.

Diarrhea recipes for children: Parch ½ pint of rice until perfectly brown, then boil it down as is usually done and eat it slowly, and it is claimed will stop bad diarrhea in a few hours. An old German-Czech recipe: Measure 2 small cups of flour. Put in skillet on stove under low fire. Keep stirring until a light brown. Allow to cool. When cool put in a jar. Take a tablespoonful, put in small cup and a little water to make a paste. Either take this as is or put on a piece of bread. Take every 3 hours if the diarrhea is persistent. A Swiss recipe: Apply to the abdomen a towel which has been wetted with warm water. Renew frequently. Feed child with porridge of warm oatmeal.

Worm recipes for children: Have the child drink fresh juice of carrots. Fresh ripe bilberries or strawberries are given to children with worms in folk practice. Onion recipes: Put minced onions in layers with a little sugar and allow to steep overnight. Give juice in teaspoonful doses. Or: Cook onions in milk, give teaspoonful in the morning and at night.

COLDS

Eating a little fresh parsley greens everyday is said to help prevent colds. *See Parsley in Part I.*

An infusion made with dried raspberries in boiling water is prized in Russian home practice as a diaphoretic. The infusion is taken hot upon retiring.

A university team found that students who ate apples had fewer colds and upper respiratory difficulties than those who did not eat them. Apple peel is rich in vitamin C but must be chewed thoroughly to derive benefits.

Germans put a little paprika in tea or corn whiskey as a preventive against colds. Paprika is very rich in vitamin C.

Head cold and polypus are claimed to be cured with lemon juice when used as a nasal rinse.

Head colds may often be averted if one keeps the nose well filled with the vapor of crushed garlic at the first symptoms. To many, the cure is probably worse than the disease.

CONSTIPATION

An apple or 2 eaten every morning for breakfast, without other food or beverage, will help regulate bowel action. The apple with peel must be slowly and thoroughly chewed. Fruit should not be chilled. Always clean apples thoroughly to remove poisonous chemical sprays and enhancing agents.

Another source recommended baked apples for sluggish stools. Sugar, salt, and butter should not be used on baked apples.

This writer found the Rome type apple, one eaten before retiring, very effective as a laxative. *See Apple Diet; also see Apple article in Part I.*

A tablespoonful of sultana raisins, taken regularly before evening meals, softens stools.

Figs cooked in milk make a useful drink for costive invalids.

Sauerkraut eaten raw is an excellent laxative. Heat destroys valuable enzymes and the kraut is then only useful for its fiber and bulk. Well chewed raw cabbage also has laxative properties.

Cooked rhubarb stalks have a laxative action. As rhubarb contains oxalic acid it should be avoided by those who suffer from arthritis, rheumatism and gout.

A few whole seeds of mustard (white or black) swallowed without chewing often helps bowel movements.

Chicken gumbo soup made with okra is a mild laxative. Okra contains an indigestible residue which forms bulk in the digestive tract.

Ripe bananas are beneficial in regulating too frequent bowel action.

Prunes have gentle laxative properties. They soften and add fiber, bulk and fluid to the stools.

A small glass of fresh pumpkin or squash juice before breakfast is an effective laxative.

Carrots well chewed aid bowel action.

Excerpt from *Meals Medicinal:* "Onions are helpful against constipation, by reason mainly of their abundant cellulose, which gives intestinal momentum."

An old family recipe book states that roasted Spanish onion eaten at bedtime is a good laxative.

COUGHING. *Also see Bronchial.*
Minced fresh horseradish root mixed with honey and sugar is a home remedy for coughing and to loosen phlegm in catarrh, asthma and lung congestion. Dr. H. Wallnöfer of Austria wrote that horseradish root has antibiotic properties.

Add honey to finely chopped garlic. Take a teaspoonful every hour or as needed . . . or as can be tolerated.

Cook lightly minced leeks in a small quantity of milk. After this has cooled add enough honey to make a syrup. Take teaspoonful as needed.

A very popular folk recipe for coughing "of all kinds": Mince 2 onions very fine and put a spoonful in a cup; sprinkle sugar over the onions, then add another layer in the same way and allow it to stand overnight. Take a teaspoonful at a time. The recipe also is used for head colds; "buzzing" in ears, numbness and dizziness.

A much older recipe recommends onions and sugar should be well cooked. It is used for bad coughs and hoarseness due to colds.

Raw onions are occasionally taken with advantage as an expectorant by elderly persons affected with winter cough.

Make a syrup of the juice of black currant mixed with honey. Take in teaspoonful doses. The syrup is specially esteemed for whooping cough.

Dr. W. J. Fischer, author of *Heilpflanzen der Heimat,* recommended the heated juice of black currants for chronic rhinitis and whooping cough.

A delicious jelly made with ripe black currants is used for whooping cough. For medicinal use, the jelly is thinned with a little hot water. Black currant fruits are rich in vitamin C and minerals.

A syrup made with figs cooked in water is commonly used in Europe for coughs in children. Another popular children's recipe is made by cooking equal parts of figs with St. John's bread. A recipe children do not relish is made by cooking equal parts of St. John's bread (without seeds) with sliced onions in water.

Dry cough: Save the water which potatoes with skins were boiled in; sweeten with sugar or honey. Take spoonful as needed. Another: Lightly cook sliced onions with wine vinegar. Strain and add an equal amount of honey to the infusion. Take spoonful hourly.

Cooked oatmeal sweetened with honey eases coughs.

The juice of black radish mixed with honey is a folk remedy for coughing.

Carrot juice in honey or sweetened with sugar is used for cough and the prepared mixture is sold in many German Apothekes.

An excellent syrup for coughs of cold or whooping cough is made with the liquid from thoroughly boiled red beet roots and sugar. Syrup of turnip root is made and used in the same way.

DEBILITY & CONVALESCENCE

Oats are the most nutritious of all cereals, and one of the most widely used foods for debility and convalescence. The meal is simply prepared as porridge or broth cooked in milk or water. Cooked with fruits, vegetables or nuts it makes a restorative as well as a substantial food for vegetarians. Malt made with barley also has high nutritive value and is used with other foods in debilitating conditions. Malt extracts are of value in the case of persons of feeble digestive powers when given with such foods as porridge, gruel, bread with milk, or arrowroot, which they help to digest. *See chapters Barley and Oats in Part I.*

Avocado pear contains more easily digested protein than all other fruits and up to 25 percent fat, plus vitamin B complex and fat-soluble vitamin A. The fruit is an excellent addition in salads and diets for convalescence when permitted.

Ripe bananas eaten raw, or in desserts, puddings, salads, etc. are nutritious and strengthening as well as easily digested. They may be eaten by infants and people with ulcers or colitis and diabetics on low sodium diets. Bananas are also a good source of potassium.

A Chinese herbal dated about 1289 prescribed bananas in all states of depletion and in convalescence from long illnesses.

Sweet wines in moderation are stimulating and strengthening for sickly adults, elderly and those in convalescence.

Drinking 1 or 2 cupfuls daily of fresh apple juice sweetened with honey is refreshing and beneficial.

For vitamin and mineral-rich foods see Dandelion, Parsley, Spinach and Watercress in Part I.

DIABETES MELLITUS

Soya bean is used in the diet of diabetics as its carbohydrates are less assimilable. The bean contains 20 percent fat, 40 percent protein, 2 percent lecithin and steroidsaponine. It also contains vitamins B, E and provitamin A and amino acids. Soya beans are said to contain 4 times more calories than beef.

Unrefined rolled oats are strengthening in diet for diabetics as well as for the sick, convalescent, babies and people of all ages. Oats are rich in calcium and a variety of minerals.

The tubers of Jerusalem artichoke contain inulin and levulin, carbohydrates that are not converted into sugar in the body. It is said the tubers are high in vitamins and minerals and low in calories. Jerusalem artichoke may be eaten raw, boiled, baked, in stews, soups and salads. *The Grocer's Manual* (1879) mentions tubers being pickled, used as a condiment and also fed to farm stock. The plant is related to sunflowers and grows in a wild state from southern Canada to Oklahoma and nearby areas. Plants are easily grown and tubers are offered by some nurseries.

Unsweetened red currant juice is used as a beverage in Europe for diabetics.

Professor Dr. Heupke of Austria claims cucumber juice or cucumbers eaten in salads tends to lower sugar in blood.

The dried pods of kidney beans (*Phaseolus vulgaris*) without the seeds are still much used in Europe in strong decoction as a diuretic to lower blood sugar levels of diabetics.

Asparagus is recommended in the diet of diabetics because of its low carbohydrate content.

A doctor from Udaipur, India, reported fried onions lower blood sugar in diabetes; adding some garlic juice is even better. The experiment was tried on 4 groups of diabetic rabbits. The sugar-lowering effect of the onion and garlic was found to be as good as that of tolbutamide, a standard diabetes treatment drug.

DIARRHEA & DYSENTERY

An authoritative Austrian source advised fresh or cooked apples without peel or core for diarrhea, dysentery and vomiting. Pectin is an important constituent of apples. Some years ago bacteriologists found that broth containing pectin becomes sterile after 48 hours of incubation.

Wild crab apples abound with tannin and are highly astringent. Dr. Fernie wrote that they are helpful against some forms of chronic diarrhea.

An infusion made with dried bilberries (*Vaccinium myrtillus*) is very effective in diarrhea. Boil 3 dessertspoonfuls of the dried fruit in 1 pint of water; cook about 10 minutes. Allow to steep until cool, then strain. Dose: 1 wineglassful for adults, 3 or 4 times daily. The dried berries may be chewed instead of brewing. An English source adds that bilberry jam is excellent against diarrhea, with putridity, and flatulence from bacterial fermentation. Bilberries contain the glucosides ericolin, arbutin and myrtillin plus tannin, sugar, pectin and vacciniin. The berries are very flavorful, high in nutritional value for vitamins and minerals and official in German pharmacopoeia. Bilberries are also known as whortleberries and are native to the British Isles and many parts of Europe and northern Asia. The berries are much like our native blueberries and huckleberries and probably have similar properties.

An astringent syrup made by boiling quince fruit in water is used for diarrhea. The fruit is rich in pectin and the kernels contain more than 22 percent mucilage, a constituent that is soothing to the intestinal tract.

An old English *Domestic Dictionary* states, "The grated rind of the pomegranate is said to have been found a sovereign remedy for diarrhea and dysentery, when all other things have failed."

A syrup made with the strained juice of blackberries with sugar is good for children with diarrhea. Give 2 to 4 tablespoonfuls daily. Strained blackberry jam or jelly is also useful.

Blackberry brandy in moderate doses is an excellent (and tasty) medicine for adults with diarrhea.

Mashed fresh huckleberries steeped with honey for a month or more is a highly regarded household remedy for children with diarrhea. Dose: One teaspoon hourly.

Vitamin-rich black currants are much used in the diet for people suffering from diarrhea in northern Europe and Asia where the bush is grown in gardens and found in the wild.

Bananas have long been noted for their efficacy in correcting the fluxes to which Europeans are often subject on their first coming into the West Indies. Bananas are rich in potassium and help replace this important element that is lost in vomiting, diarrhea and dysentery.

Peasants used the finely pulverized seeds of grapes for diarrhea and dysentery.

In Europe dehydrated carrot or apple stirred in water is used in orthodox practice for diarrhea in young children. The pectin constituent of either carrot or apple is effective against diarrhea, especially for the tender and sensitive intestinal tract of children.

Cinnamon sticks steeped in red wine are an "ausgezeichnetes" (outstanding) agent for adults with diarrhea or dysentery when taken in small doses. From the same herbal: Eat well cooked rice with a light dash of cinnamon.

A soothing home remedy for diarrhea: Boil rice in plenty of water or milk for about ½ hour; strain through a cloth. Drink a cupful of the liquid at a time as often as desired or needed. Abstain from other liquids. Rice liquid may be sweetened with honey. The recipe also is very good for chronic diarrhea.

Oatmeal cooked with milk is very soothing to intestinal tract in diarrhea or dysentery.

Unrefined barley cooked with milk is particularly good for diarrhea caused by adulterated or spoiled foods.

DIURETICS

Diuretics are used to increase the flow of urine. The following food and beverage plants have diuretic tendencies: Asparagus shoots, celery seed, coffee, leeks, melons of all sorts, onions, parsley leaves or root, parsnip greens, root and seed, string bean pods (no seeds), tea, watercress and many other less active food plants.

Eating a plenteous onions, cooked or raw, in diet helps increase urine excretion and for this reason is useful in dropsy, retained urine, and kidney disturbances.

Leeks are both very wholesome, and in a cooked state are a mild diuretic, but they have a much stronger effect if taken raw. One of the best diuretics for domestic use is the fibres from the bottom of the root, washed, and steeped for a week in gin; about ½ wine-glass to be taken at night in a tumbler of water.

Old English recipe: The water wherein turnip roots are boiled will increase the flow of urine.

Grated fresh horseradish root thoroughly mixed with butter is rubbed over the bladder area to stimulate urine action. This is an old European folk recipe. Another: Rub the loins with sliced onions.

DROPSY, early stages

From an old home medical book: "Drink 1 or 2 cups a day an infusion or decoction made of parsley root especially following scarlet fever, retained urine, painful urination and gonorrhea."

Other sources recommend the parsley greens or roots for diuretic action. Parsley seeds are powerfully diuretic but not recommended for home use. *See Parsley in Part I.*

Watercress is used in diets for dropsy in home practice.

The dried pods (without seeds) of kidney beans boiled in water and taken a cupful or less at a time increase excretion of urine and helps prevent uric acid. Kidney beans are also called French or climbing purple-podded kidney bean. The seeds of kidney beans contain the alkaloid phaseoline which is destroyed when cooked.

Further information on kidney beans is given under heading KIDNEY & BLADDER.

The decoction made with celery seeds in water is commonly used as a diuretic for dropsy.

The infusion made with water and parsnip seed is used to drain excessive water from the body.

An old German recipe advised eating cooked asparagus and drinking the water in which it was cooked. *See Asparagus in Part I.*

The American Dispensatory by John King, M.D. (8th ed., 1872) prescribed horseradish root for dropsy. It stated: "An infusion of the root in cider, and drank as warm as could be borne in large quantities and freely, the patient being warmly covered up, has caused copious diuresis and diaphoresis, and cured the disease in a few weeks; the operation being repeated nightly, or as the strength of the patient would permit."

EAR

The juice of white cabbage with equal parts of wine dropped in the ears, is used among peasants to improve hearing.

Roasted sliced onions applied to the ear as warm as can be tolerated relieves earache.

Dr. Fernie advised: "When there is running fetid discharge from the ear, or when an abscess is first threatened, with pain, heat, and swelling, the hot poultice of roasted onions will be found very soothing, and will do much to mitigate the pain; or, a clove of garlic, stripped of the outer skin, and cut in the form of a blunt cone, if thrust gently into the aching side, will quickly assuage the pain."

When earache is caused by a cold put a few drops of garlic or onion juice in warm olive oil and put into the ear.

ENERGY FRUITS & VEGETABLES

Bananas, cabbage, carrots, dates, figs, grapes, honey, oatmeal, onions, peas, prunes, raisins, soybeans, spinach, strawberries, and black currants are considered energy foods.

EYES

A modern German source states the leaves of chervil have a beneficial action against ophthalmia. The herb contains a volatile oil with methylchavicol as the main component and the leaves contain the flavon glycoside apiin. Chervil acts as a stimulant, mild diuretic and blood purifier taken as an infusion. Fresh chervil is much used in France in soups, stews and salads. *See Spring Cure.*

The flavorful fruit of black currants are widely used in Europe for their high nutritional value as well as for their curative properties. It is said to increase vision capability and is a protective against vessel disturbances.

Peter Mertes' book *Heilpflanzen* (1936) gives this old fashioned recipe: "Onions cooked in milk and honey serves as an eyewash."

Sugar water is a home remedy used to remove foreign matter from the eye.

A Nürnberg recipe: Apply cold water to the eyelids, eyebrows and temples several times daily to strengthen eyes.

FEET

Onions cooked with vinegar are applied to corns. The application is renewed several times. Another: Apply a slice of garlic to the corn and renew application.

Apply the juice of lemon on chafed feet. The application is also good for rough hands.

A fresh piece of lemon peel fastened on a corn at night is said to cure it in a few days. Application should be renewed each night.

FEVER

A strengthening and refreshing beverage is made with red raspberry syrup or raspberry vinegar added to lemonade. Red raspberry syrup is made by cooking 7 parts of the strained fruit juice with 10 parts sugar. Raspberry vinegar is made with 1 part of raspberry syrup with 2 parts of wine vinegar.

The juice of blackberries in water makes a refreshing beverage for fevers. The berries are a good source of iron, calcium and other minerals, plus vitamins, especially vitamin C.

The juice of red currant fruit mixed with water and sweetened with honey makes a cooling and agreeable beverage for children with miliary fever.

Drink the cooled decoction made with water and dried apple peels. Or eat apples with peel cut into small pieces. It will quench thirst.

An old French physician claimed that the bacillus of typhoid fever cannot live beyond a very short time in pure apple juice;

he therefore advised persons residing where the drinking water is not above suspicion to mix cider therewith before imbibing it.

Dr. Fernie wrote that the fresh juice of bilberry (*Vaccinium myrtillus*) is antidotal to the bacillus of typhoid fever, as well as to some other kindred bacilli, generally killing these within 12 hours after reaching them within the intestines. Neither the acid gastric juice of the stomach, nor the alkaline contents of the bowels, will interfere with such germicidal action, which extends down to the lowest part of the alimentary canal. Likewise this fruit confers sure benefit against dysentery by its destructive power on bacilli.

An excellent beverage in fever: Take a handful of unrefined barley; boil in water until seed shells separate; strain and add the juice of ½ lemon and enough honey to sweeten. Drink a mouthful at a time. *See Barley in Part I.*

Rolled oats cooked into a watery solution is a home recipe for hectic fever.

FLU

In Europe an extract made with garlic is a very popular household remedy for flu as well as a remedy for assorted other symptoms. The extract is made by steeping ½ lb. of chopped garlic in 1 qt. of brandy for 2 weeks or more in the sun or a warm place. The extract should be kept well corked and in a dark brown bottle. The garlic may be allowed to remain or strained from the brandy. It is said the extract will keep about 1 year. Ten to 15 drops may be taken an hour before each meal for adults.

Another home recipe: To the juice of 1 lemon, add 3 teaspoonfuls of honey, 4 teaspoonfuls of rum, mix this in a glass of water as hot as can be tolerated. Drink before retiring.

Preventive measures: Drink the juice of raw sauerkraut. Eat black currant fruits or drink the juice. Drink the juice of ½ lemon with a little water in the morning, another ½ at noon and again before retiring.

GALL BLADDER

In European folk practice the juice of fresh radish root (black or white) is used to cure or palliate gall bladder disturbances. The treatment generally is taken over a 1 or 2 week period. The patient begins with 2 or 3 oz. of radish juice and increases the amounts each day until 4 or 5 oz. are taken, then gradually reducing the dosage after the middle of the treatment. The radish "cure" has been used for ages. Beneficial results have been claimed.

Another source states minced radishes with olive oil and a little lemon stimulates appetite and benefits the gall bladder.

An Austrian herbal claims folks should eat an ample amount of black radish roots to prevent gall and kidney stone formation.

Another source adds the Japanese use black radish as a prophylactic against many kinds of known and unknown infections.

Radish roots, especially the black variety, contain raphanin, an antibiotic.

Radishes should not be salted when used for medicinal purposes. *See Radish in Part I.*

Fresh grape juice taken like the grape cure diet once or twice a year is believed in Tyrol to help prevent formation of gallstones, kidney and bladder stones.

Garlic used generously in the diet is claimed to work favorably on bile. (Always use foods in moderation, especially if not accustomed to generous amounts.)

Olive oil is used in the treatment of gall stones and aids in promoting normal bile flow, according to a French doctor.

GOITER, Simple

In goiter-prone areas, such as remote regions cut off by mountain ranges from the sea, iodine is often deficient in foods grown in these environments. The following plant sources usually supply ample iodine: Swiss chard, turnip and mustard greens, summer squash, cucumbers, spinach, asparagus, kale and watercress. Kelp, a seaweed, contains far more natural iodine as well as minerals than any land plant used as food. Kelp tablets are available in Health Food Stores.

In a U.S. Public Health report it was revealed that simple goiter was most prevalent in all states north of Arizona and New Mexico and all states surrounding the Great Lakes region.

GRAPE DIET

The Grape Diet originated some 2,500 years ago to aid high Roman officials and the wealthy to mend their digestive tracts impaired by overindulgences and debauchery. Through the centuries the custom was accepted by many health-minded people as well as prescribed by many European physicians for a variety of ailments including chronic constipation, enlarged congested livers, obesity and where uric acid is present in excess in the blood.

Grapes grown in the region of Merano, Italy, are considered most beneficial because of the high radioactive concentrations in water and soil of this particular area. Wines of this region are said to be extremely aromatic.

The following (with variations or modifications depending upon the condition of the patient) appears to be most popular among folk seeking benefits from the grape regimen. Only the pulp (no skins or seeds) of the fully ripe fruit is eaten and complete fasting from all foods and beverages is considered most effective. The diet is taken 1 or 2 days several times in a 2-week period. The diet consists of eating 4 to 6 pounds of grape pulp daily. Even larger quantities are sometimes taken depending, of course, on the sex, age and weight of the person. When total fasting could not be tolerated the patient ate a small piece of whole wheat bread and drank a little chamomile or linden flower tea an hour after eating the grape pulp. Lunch and evening meals, taken an hour after more grape pulp is consumed, consisted of small portions of nourishing foods. Fats, meats, salads, white bread, bakery goods, spices, vinegar, wines, beer, soft drinks, milk and water are strictly avoided. Medical supervision is recommended in total fasting diet. Disciples of the grape diet believe it not only cures some conditions but also helps prepare the body for rigors of winter. Grape pulp contains fructose and glucose sugars readily assimilated and a source of quick energy. The insoluble lignin and high water contents of grape pulp have a decided laxative effect. The diet is not recommended for everyone as it often has adverse effects causing diarrhea and swelling of the gums from excessive acid.

In Europe other fruits are also used in various cures lasting from 4 to 6 weeks. Apples, pears, oranges, lemons, in fact almost all fruits have been vaunted as cures. Various methods are followed, but the basis of all is a restricted diet with an abundance of fruit. The diets are used in the same conditions for which the grape cure has been prescribed.

Common sense should be used with diet cures. If they achieve no benefits there is no sense in continuing. Moderation usually is best in any regimen.

HAIR
An old German book on healing herbs states that a strong decoction of celery seed is used as a wash to remove dandruff and to strengthen hair.

Another: Steep 4 or 5 finely minced garlic cloves in hard liquor for 10 days in the sun. Strain and rub scalp with liquid twice a day. To reduce the garlic odor dab scalp with a little oil of rosemary.

A folk recipe recommends applying the juice of garlic to the scalp to stimulate hair growth.

A recipe from Nürnberg: In a pint of brandy steep slices of a large onion and allow to steep 2 weeks. Strain and add 2 parts water. Rub on scalp once a day.

Recipe to check falling hair, providing there are no scalp or other troubles: Massage scalp thoroughly with olive oil before retiring. Wear a slumber cap and shampoo in the morning. Continue until falling is checked.

Good results with rolled oat diet have been claimed for hair growth following pathological diseases.

Crushed oats fed with hay to horses is said to give the hair of the animal a lustrous sheen.

See HERBAL RECIPES by this author for other valuable hair recipes.

HEADACHE
An old German doctor's recipe: Lay fresh crushed parsley roots upon a cloth and hold to the head; renew application with fresh roots when it becomes warm.

From the same source: A foot bath made with powdered mustard is "an active agent" against headaches and inflammation of the eyes.

Grated fresh horseradish root held to the back of the neck is said to relieve headaches. A very old recipe states: "The most excruciating head and toothache has often been suddenly dispelled by applying fresh horseradish shavings or bruised garlic between 2 fine pieces of muslin, to the bend of both arms or hams."

A Nürnberg recipe: Drink a cupful of hot strong coffee in which the juice of ½ lemon has been added.

From the same source: If headache is caused by alcohol, eat 1 or 2 apples, chewing thoroughly.

Stomach or gastric headaches are usually caused by overloading the stomach or eating food that does not agree, such as fat meat, greasy gravies, starch food, pastry, etc. Drinking water as hot as can be tolerated often gives quick relief.

Headache caused by constipation generally causes a dull heavy feeling, sometimes dizziness, a bad taste in the mouth and drowsiness so that work goes hard. Good stool action will relieve this type headache. *See Constipation.*

For nervous headache see Tension.

For menstrual headache see Menses.

HEART

A French tonic recipe: Add a heaping teaspoonful of pulverized dried apple peels to a cupful of boiling water; allow to steep until cool. Drink frequently. Sweeten with honey.

A chemical found in ripe bananas (norepinephrine) has been used in the treatment of heart. Bananas alone will not cure heart ailments but they are considered a health food for all age groups.

Onions are reputed to strengthen heart action according to *Das Gewürzbuch.*

Another German source states that regular use of garlic hinders the possibility of cardiac infarction while a French source claims eating 2 apples a day is a preventive measure.

A 1974 news item states that two English doctors reported garlic helped "thin" the blood in ten patients on a fatty diet and could be helpful in preventing heart disease. The English reporter added that it will also get you a seat on a crowded bus . . . worth trying these days.

All heart conditions as well as all other serious conditions require professional care.

INTESTINAL DISORDERS

Thoroughly ripened grated fresh apples, without peel or core, taken as sole diet for several days, is claimed to be superior for acute or chronic intestinal catarrh and coli bacillus infections. Sugar and fluid intake are strictly avoided. Austrian authorities believed either the raw or cooked apples may be used for acute or chronic catarrh. The same source adds that fruit or juice of blackberries may be used for intestinal catarrh.

Many Germans believed there is nothing better than raw sauerkraut for its enzyme action upon putrid fermentation in the bowels. Enzymes are destroyed when kraut is cooked. Two dessertspoonfuls of the raw kraut are generally taken per day. If kraut is too acrid, eat a little whole wheat bread with it.

Raw white cabbage is also claimed of benefit for intestinal disturbances. *See Cabbage in Part I.*

Garlic and onions contain allicine, an agent that inhibits colon bacteria causing indigestion, fermentation and putrefaction of the stomach and colon contents. Garlic is most useful when digestive functions have been decreased or enfeebled by age. A home recipe for using garlic for fermentation and putrid dyspepsia: Peel a small clove of garlic and allow it to steep by stirring in a glass of cold water that has been sterilized. Strain off the clove, take a teaspoonful hourly. *See Garlic in Part I.*

Fine sliced onions boiled in milk is a home remedy for colic or abdominal pains. Drink the milk while it is warm.

To alleviate abdominal cramps: Drink a cupful of warm infusion made like ordinary tea of dried parsley greens or root.

Dr. Carl Böhme recommended ripe black currant fruit steeped in brandy for stomach and abdominal complaints.

A wine made of bilberries (whortleberries) is used for inflammation of the mucous membrane of the colon. Bilberries, native of Europe and Asia, resemble American blueberries.

A well known Austrian herbalist believes carrots are one of the best agents for putrefaction or inflammation of the colon. An easily digested meal for stomach and colon ailments is made with chopped carrots cooked in water until made into a thick porridge, an equal portion (or less) of oxtail soup is added to the strained carrot porridge. Plain cooked and strained carrots are much used for infants and children with colon and stomach ailments. Neither the porridge or soup should be salted.

INSOMNIA
In the evening drink 1 glass of lukewarm water with 25 drops of extract of garlic and sweeten with 1 or 2 teaspoons of honey. *See recipe under FLU for garlic extract.*

A warm dish of cooked rolled oats or oatmeal eaten just before retiring is a harmless soporific for elderly folks.

At bedtime drink a warm infusion made of dill seeds. Steep 1 teaspoonful of the seeds in a cupful of boiling water; strain when lukewarm.

A rustic recipe: Rub the nap of the neck and foot soles with raw garlic just before retiring.

In homeopathic practice an extract made from fresh white or black radish roots is used for sleeplessness as well as restlessness.

An apple slowly and thoroughly chewed before retiring often brings quiet sleep.

Liqueur recipe for nightcap: Crush fully ripe black currant fruit and add to a good brandy. Allow it to steep 7 or 8 days—during the day in sunshine. Strain and allow to stand another week. Add sugar syrup to taste. Drink jiggerful upon retiring. Crushed fresh peppermint added with the black currant in brandy makes a good stomachic.

Recent tests conducted by the Department of Psychiatry at Edinburgh University revealed that a hot milky drink before bedtime induces longer and more restful sleep.

Another source advises taking ¼ teaspoonful of nutmeg gratings and a pinch of red pepper in ½ glass of hot milk in which 2 teaspoonfuls of honey have been dissolved.

Eat a dish of warm boiled onions before retiring. Frank Buckland once said: "If I am much pressed with work and feel that I am not disposed to sleep, I eat 2 or 3 small onions and their effect is magical."

See American Folk Medicine *by this author for other insomnia recipes.*

KIDNEY & BLADDER, Also see Diuretics
The fruit or juice of black currants is much used in Europe for retention of urine, gravel, cystitis, nephritis, renal colic and dropsy. Father Kneipp especially recommended black currants for the elderly. For centuries they were regarded as an elixir of

life. The medicinal properties of this fruit are still highly regarded in home and orthodox practices.

A domestic recipe for pain in the bladder and bedwetting: Put enough corn kernels in barley water to make a thick mixture. Allow it to stand until kernels become soft. Heat the mixture to a degree it can be tolerated and apply to the area of the bladder as a poultice.

The application of crushed fresh parsley to the bladder area is used in folk practice to palliate inflammation of that organ. Another: Drink a decoction made of parsley root or the dehydrated greens.

A simple and often effective remedy for cystitis and retention of urine: Simmer a handful of leeks in enough olive oil to cover. Apply warm to the area of the bladder.

Pain from retained urine: Heat a cloth bag filled with sliced onions and apply to the lower abdomen. Reheat bag repeatedly as it cools off.

A decoction made with dried watermelon seeds has an old reputation for being beneficial for kidney trouble.

The juice of cranberries is often recommended for cystitis or burning of urine. The berries contain the glucoside vacciin, organic acids, pectin, iron, and vitamin A, B_1, B_2, and C.

Cooked asparagus shoots or spears, as well as the water in which it is prepared, is commonly used for ailments of the kidney organs. The vegetable is recommended in diet for people with kidney trouble.

Asparagus roots are used in professional practice as a strong diuretic for acute or chronic cystopyelitis with no after effects when properly used, according to a former head Physician of the University of Munich Clinic.

French grandmothers prescribed a broth made of leeks, milk and potatoes for inflamed kidneys. The broth should not be salted or peppered.

Apple peels, well chewed, increase secretion of uric acid. (*Also see Grape Cure.*) French folk recipe for uremic poisoning: Steep an ounce of leek rootlets in a quart of good white wine. Keep bottle in sunny location for 10 days. Drink a wine glass each morning.

In home practice 5 or 6 teaspoonfuls of fresh mashed huckleberries mixed with honey is used for common bladder troubles.

European folk recipe used to promote urine and ease the pain of kidney stones: Gather and dry the leaves of parsnip when plant is in bloom. To a pint of water add 2 or 3 tablespoonfuls of crushed dried leaves and boil about 10 minutes. Strain and drink a wineglassful 3 times a day. The root is also used as a diuretic. Take 2 or 3 tablespoonfuls of the minced fresh root 3 times a day.

Celery has diuretic properties and is used in diet for bladder ailments. An excellent recipe: Cut celery stalks in ½-inch (or so) lengths. Cook in chicken soup until stalks are tender.

From *Heilkräuter und Arzneipflanzen* by G. Fischer, 1966: "The dehydrated kidney bean pods without the seeds are used for all types of dropsical conditions as a result of heart or kidney ailments, kidney inflammation, after scarlet fever, diphtheria, typhus, as with articular rheumatism and gout, with albuminous urine in pregnancy, by water accumulation as a result from a single organ, finally by all illnesses of the urinary passages, acute and chronic from the kidneys to the urethra from gravel to stone formation. No other [plant] agent is capable of checking and loosening the formation of uric acid than cooked kidney bean pods. Dosage for 1 day: Soak 4 or 5 ounces of dehydrated bean pods (without seeds) in 1 quart of water, boil, then simmer down to 1 pint. Strain when cold. Drink small draughts through the day."

From Dr. W. T. Fernie's *Meals Medicinal:* "Medical testimony goes to show that in countries and districts where natural cider is the common beverage, stone in the bladder is quite unknown. A series of enquiries among the doctors of Normandy (which is a great apple country, where cider is the chief if not the sole drink) has established the fact that not a single case of the nature in question had been met with there throughout forty years: so that it may be fairly credited that the habitual use of natural unsweetened cider serves to keep held in solution materials which are otherwise liable to be separated, and deposited in a sedimentary form by the kidneys."

LIVER
The juice of white cabbage is used in Europe for the treatment of liver damage; especially when caused by alcoholism.

Horseradish stimulates liver action and helps the digestion of fatty meats.

A 1952 report states that the Russians treated epidemic infectious hepatitis with horseradish root. The botanical promotes the flow of bile, stimulates the appetite and helps shorten the duration of the disease. Horseradish root must be fresh. Heat dissipates its therapeutic properties.

The French believe that the liberal use of fresh or cooked carrots in salads, soups, stews, etc. is of benefit to the liver as well as for general health. The raw juice of carrots is very popular among health zealots.

Dr. Fernie wrote that the acids of apples are of signal use for men of sedentary habits whose livers are torpid; they serve to eliminate from the body noxious matters which would, if retained, make the brain heavy and dull.

Daily use of apples benefits the liver and indirectly helps general health.

Watercress is considered by an Austrian herbalist the "beste Speise" for liver ailments.

Grossmutter and Grossvater were firm believers that eating radishes of all kinds was beneficial to the liver and gall bladder. Both white and so-called black roots were eaten raw. A syrup made with sugar added to the raw juice was also used. *See Radish in Part I.*

Turmeric, a spice used in mustards, pickles, curries, sauces, etc., is an old and highly esteemed medicinal in India. In modern times it has become a specific agent for liver and gall disturbances according to Dr. G. Boros of Switzerland.

The gold colored roots of turmeric contain up to 5 percent volatile oil, a bitter, resin and the light sensitive coloring matter curcumin. In Indian home practice the mild infusion of the dried root is taken in small doses.

LUNGS

The fruit of black currant or huckleberries is used in Europe in diet for inflammation of the lungs.

Onions fried in lard and rubbed on the chest as hot as can be tolerated helps loosen phlegm in the lungs.

Tightness in chest: Upon retiring take a dessertspoonful of minced horseradish root mixed with honey. Or take a teaspoonful hourly of onion juice sweetened with sugar.

A folk recipe for inflammation of the lungs: Finely grate 2 horseradish roots; then add a little milk to make a paste. Apply to the area of pain, allowing 2 minutes for children and 5 minutes for adults. The inflammation is claimed to leave within half a day. It is important that the patient remains in bed 2 days to avoid reoccurrence.

In Europe parsnip root is used in the diet of consumptives. The root contains water, nitrogenous substance, fat, sugar, pectin, carbohydrate, minerals and vitamins.

Carrots cooked in milk are also believed to be a strengthening food for consumptives and weakness. Cooked carrots are exceptionally rich in provitamin A (carotene).The root also contains glucose, sucrose, pectin, iron, calcium and other minerals.

MEMORY, Weak

Equal parts of carrot juice with milk is claimed in folk practice to strengthen the memory of old people. The mixture is easily digested and must be taken daily.

Drink 1 or 2 cups daily of rosemary tea well sweetened with honey. Rosemary tea is made like ordinary tea. Melisse tea is also highly recommended.

A diet of strawberries is believed by some Europeans an aid for weak memory.

The wife of a well known American president ate chocolate covered garlic pills to stimulate memory. A German physician wrote that garlic dilates vessels and relieves tension of the brain.

A Künzle recipe: Cook in wine finely chopped parsley root and greens. Strain when cool. Drink ½ wineglassful morning and night.

Dr. Tobias Venner, an old-time English physician, advised the universities that green ginger is good for the memory. Green ginger refers to fresh ginger. The candied spice, made from the fresh root, probably may be used.

Ginger is an agreeable stimulant and formerly the infusion was very popular as a stomach warmer for the elderly. The infusion is not boiled as heat drives off the volatile oils which are their active principles. The dried root also deoxidizes and rapidly loses its qualities when exposed to air and as it ages.

MENSES

Two teaspoonfuls of fresh horseradish root steeped in a little red wine is a stimulus for menstrual period.

An infusion made with water and parsley roots or greens often alleviates menstrual disturbances (amenorrhea or dysmenorrhea).

A weak infusion made like ordinary tea of celery seed is an old-fashioned home remedy for menstrual troubles. The tea is taken warm.

An infusion of carrot seed is also used as an emmenagogue.

A very popular recipe when ladies had to refer to home medical guides for their ills: When menses were stopped or caused cramps by colds, drink freely of the warm ginger tea before retiring. Ginger tea should not be boiled as heat dissipates its volatile and medicinal properties.

MENTAL DEPRESSION

Ripe bananas contain two important chemicals which are powerful in their pure state but harmless to humans of all ages because of nature's blend with many other plant constituents. The chemicals serotonin and norepinephrine contained in bananas are necessary for the normal function of the brain. Authorities believe a high level of the chemicals is desirable to prevent mental depression. *See Motherhood for banana constituents.*

Wine is a most useful medicinal, when discreetly used, for nursing homes to enliven depressing mental attitudes of elderly. Pleasant moods ease nurse's duties too.

An Austrian recipe for mental exhaustion: Pour a pint of boiling hot water over an apple (with peel) that has been cut into small pieces. Allow to steep about an hour and add 2 or 3 teaspoonfuls of honey. Eat apple pieces, then drink the infusion.

Dr. Fernie wrote that sultana raisins, when stewed, will recruit and revive the tired body and the jaded mind.

MOTHERHOOD

In Europe mothers having trouble breast feeding their babies ate a gruel made of unrefined barley meal cooked with milk. The breast milk is said to be rich and agreeable to the infant. A little fennel seed is sometimes added to the barley. Fennel has a reputation as a "friend of the stomach." *See Barley in Part I.*

Cooked carrots or malt beer are often recommended for nursing mothers.

Nursing mothers may increase their milk production by drinking warm infusions made with crushed dill seeds. Steep a teaspoonful in a cupful of boiling water. Strain when warm. Sweeten if desired.

Ancient Athenian physicians prescribed cabbage for young nursing mothers in belief their babies would grow lusty and strong.

Germans regard pea soup as very beneficial to women in childbed. Peas are an excellent plant source of protein, iron, phosphorous, potassium, niacin and vitamins A, B_1, B_2, and C. The well balanced constituents makes peas an excellent food for the tender age of children and the sensitive period of pregnancy.

From John Gerard's 1536 Herbal: "Bananas nourisheth the child in the mothers wombe, and stirreth to generation."

Ripe bananas contain significant amounts of phosphorus, potassium and other minerals and a fair source of vitamins A, B_1, B_2,

C and niacin. Having a high proportion of easily assimilable sugars, it is a good food for energy and to help relieve fatigue.

Avocado pear is excellent in diet during pregnancy when calories need not be controlled. The fruit contains more protein than any other fruit and up to 25 percent of fat. A hundred grams of avocado contains 218 calories.

A folk recipe to ease childbirth: Apply 1 or 2 handfuls of fresh parsley greens to the navel for a period before delivery.

A commonly used recipe in Europe for albumin in urine during pregnancy is to drink freely an infusion (made like ordinary tea) of the dried pods (no seeds) of kidney beans or string beans.

MOUTH, THROAT, TEETH

Honey mixed with water is used for a gargle to relieve dryness of the mouth and throat. Levulose, the sugar found in honey, increases the secretion of saliva, thus helps relieve thirst, and facilitates swallowing.

A fig split open and applied hot against gum-boils or other similar suppurative gatherings will afford ease and promote maturation of the abscess.

Hoarseness: Eat a baked apple sweetened with honey or eat a clove of garlic several times a day, if it can be tolerated.

The fresh juice of European bilberry is used as a mouth rinse. A large dose held in the mouth for some time palliates inflammation of the gums and tongue. The juice is also used as a gargle. Bilberry juice taken regularly in small doses is said to not only sweeten smoker's breath but also to discourage the habit.

A German doctor advised using only dried bilberries for medicinal uses. Three dessertspoonfuls of the dried berries are boiled in a pint of water for 10 minutes; allowed to stand until cool, then strained. The liquid is used for gargling the throat and as a mouth wash for cavities and inflamed gums.

An old English source claims fresh ripe mulberries in the form of jam or jelly is useful for sore throat.

Red raspberry vinegar made with 1 part fruit juice and 2 parts wine vinegar is a home recipe for gargle used for inflamed throat.

The juice of red currant fruits is popularly used in Europe as a mouth rinse and gargle.

A decoction made with water and dehydrated black currant fruit is reputed beneficial for inflammation of the throat. People living along the Rhine River make a flavorful jelly with black currants. When needed for sore throat the jelly is put into a glass with hot water to make a gargle.

The juice of blackberries is used in home practice for inflammation of mouth, throat or gums. A French herbal recommends blackberry jam for sore throat and irritation of the vocal cords.

A syrup of quince fruit is used for hoarseness and minor throat troubles.

Wild strawberries have more acid than the cultivated berries. The sharp juice is an excellent cleanser of the teeth, dissolving away any incrustations of tartar without injuring the enamel.

Pure lemon juice, or diluted with a little water, is useful for sore throat. An English source states: The juice of a lemon mixed with honey, in a tea cupful of hot water, is quite a specific for sore throat which is catarrhal.

Dr. Carl Böhme gave this old recipe for toothache: Make a small poultice with fresh minced horseradish root and apply it behind the ear.

Another German source recommended applying grated horse-radish root to the gum near the aching teeth.

Austrians make a gargle with powdered mustard seed, honey and water. It is said to be "sehr wirksames."

Onion juice mixed with honey is used for hoarseness and reputed to be effective for inflamed throat.

Barley water makes a soothing and effective gargle. Boil about 1½ ounces of hulled barley in a quart of water for 30 minutes. *See another barley water recipe under BARLEY in Part I.*

Foul breath recipes: To a small amount of water add minced fresh horseradish root and honey. Flush mouth thoroughly, then expectorate. Repeat several times a day.

Chew parsley greens, especially after eating garlic. Gargle with salt water or water with the juice of ½ lemon.

Whole cloves have been chewed to sweeten the breath for more than 5,000 years. Cloves have marked antiseptic powers. Chew only one clove at a time—the flavor and aroma are long lasting.

MUSCULAR PAINS
A rustic recipe: Rub aching parts with slices of raw potato or raw onions.

European peasants make a paste [a mess] with barley bran, barley meal, a little vinegar and butter. The paste is heated and applied warm to painful areas. *Also see Rheumatism and Gout.*

NERVES. *Also see Tension*
Three to 5 tablespoonfuls of onion juice mixed with honey and taken per day is believed in Europe to be "the best" nervine.

Spinach eaten in diet is believed to help strengthen nerves.

Bavarian Father Kneipp recommended fresh carrots in diets for people with nervous conditions. Dr. G. Boros of Switzerland stated that the regular use of carrots in the diet is good for nervous exhaustion and improves conditions in general.

Austrian University Dr. Heinrich Wallnöfer wrote that celery calms nerves and also is good for exhaustion. A German source states the oil derived from celery strengthens the nerves and animates the sexual powers. Six to eight drops of oil are taken twice a day in a glass of water. Old-time Germans call celery "the supply drug for deficiency ailments."

In Steiermark the bridegroom is said to eat plenty of celery before the marriage. The source did not state if the vegetable was for strength or nerves.

NERVE PAIN, Neuralgia, Neuritis, Sciatica
Germans believe eating an abundance of raw sauerkraut helps prevent sciatica.

Minced fresh horseradish root is used like mustard seed as a stimulating poultice applied for neuralgia, sciatica, cramps, etc.

An old Englsh physician advised celery tea, hot and strong (with cream and sugar, if desired), to be drunk by the teacupful 3 or 4 times in the day, so as to abate neuralgia and sciatica, which it sometimes will do very speedily.

NIGHTMARE
A homely Swiss recipe: Eat evening meal at least 2 hours before retiring; also eat less and sleep on your right side.

NOSEBLEED

To check nasal hemorrhage insert a wad of cotton wool soaked with the juice of a fresh lemon.

Dr. Carl Böhme's recipe for nose bleed: Apply a sliced onion to the nape of the neck. Or mix onion juice with vinegar and put it high into nostril.

Snuff salt water or vinegar up the nose. Another source mentions using wine vinegar for best results.

Rustic recipes: Take in each hand an onion or garlic and hold as tight as possible. This is supposed to draw the blood to the hands.

Tie a few leaves of turnip, beets, lettuce or cabbage to the neck.

Hold the hands in warm water or high over the head.

OBESITY

Instead of fattening candy bars or greasy junk foods, eat fresh carrot sticks, a few radishes, a stalk or 2 of celery or slivers of raw cabbage—even the core of raw cabbages has vitamin C. Always keep a bowlful of these items in an easily available top shelf of the refrigerator. Snackers should nip on varieties if inclined to food allergies. Fattening foods: Carbonated soft drinks (with sugar), alcoholic cocktails, beer, cream soups, gravies with flour or cream, ice cream, layer cakes, pastries, pies, sandwiches, eggs, fat meats, etc. Sedentary employment, inactivity and long sleeping hours also help add fat.

A little parsley greens eaten daily is believed by health-minded folk to help keep one thin and agile.

The Grape Diet is much used in Merano, Italy, and other vineyard regions for overweight. *See Grape Cure and Apple Diet.*

A French slimming recipe claimed to help reduce uric acid and excess fat: Before retiring eat a small dish of thinly sliced cucumbers (with peel) and season with garlic, chopped parsley, a little olive oil and a squeeze of lemon. Cucumbers must be thoroughly chewed. Diet must also be controlled.

An eighty-year-old recipe: First eat some dried apples and afterwards drink a quart of water to swell them out as a bellyful.

PHLEGM OR MUCUS
A recipe for the elderly: Add 4 tablespoonfuls of honey to 1 quart of hot water; stir thoroughly and strain through a cloth while still warm. Drink a wineglassful as needed. This simple recipe is said to be very beneficial.

Phlegm or mucus on chest: Cook chopped garlic in water and add enough sugar or honey to make a syrup. Take a teaspoonful as needed.

An excellent stimulant and solvent for abnormal mucus accumulation: To 4 ounces of finely grated horseradish add the juice of 1 lemon. It is important that only the fresh root and juice are used. Take a teaspoonful or less at a time.

Popular Old World recipe: Add 2 parts of honey to 1 part of the juice of black radish. Take a tablespoon before each meal and 1 before retiring. *See Radish in Part I.*

RESISTANCE
An author of a German folk recipe book wrote that laborers who eat plentiful of garlic have more resistance to infection when working with masses of other laborers as in large industries. It is also claimed that the garlic eaters are less likely to become fatigued as quickly as laborers who shun the smelly bulb. An interesting historical similarity: Some 5,000 years ago Pharaohs began building pyramids to perpetuate their reigns and lives

for the hereafter. It is estimated that it took about 20 years and 360,000 workers to move, almost entirely with muscle power, huge hand-hewn stone blocks fitting snugly together to form one of the Wonders of the World. The civilizations of Pharaoh's time suffered periodic plagues of typhus, pestilence and cholera. Hieroglyphic picture writings revealed that garlic and onions were rationed to the laborers employed in the construction of the pyramids. It is probable that the antiseptic, bactericidal and penetrating properties of garlic and onions provided the masses of laborers with protective resistance against infectious and catastrophic plagues as well as helped them to endure great fatigue. Garlic and onions are still grown and consumed in enormous quantities in modern Egypt.

Onions are in the same botanical family as garlic and have similar properties in a lesser degree. Other members of this most useful family are leeks, shallots, scallions, chives and many wild varieties, most all having milder properties than the common yellow onion, Allium cepa. *See Garlic and Onions in Part I.*

RHEUMATISM or GOUT
The English drink cider as it contains considerable amounts of fruit acids which are converted in the body into alkaline substances and is much used as an antacid by persons with a rheumatic tendency.

The fresh juice of carrots or tomatoes taken daily are very beneficial for rheumatism or gout. One may drink the juices alternately.

The daily use of watercress in salads without vinegar is said to help prevent gout or rheumatism.

People who eat considerable garlic generally are not afflicted with rheumatism or gout according to a German source.

Dr. Fernie's *Meals Medicinal* states that the water in which asparagus is cooked will serve to do good against rheumatism.

The fruit of black currant is a very old and popular European remedy for rheumatism or gout. Rural folks call this fruit gout-berry. The dried leaves of the bush prepared as a tea are also used for these ailments.

Dr. Ramm-Preetz wrote some years ago in regard to dehydrated string bean pods: "No other agent [plant] is capable in checking and loosening formation of uric acid in the body. For this reason the infusion is of special value for rheumatism and gout." The dried bean pods (no seeds) are infused in water like ordinary tea. Drink small draughts through the day.

A French physician wrote that fresh ripe pears eaten before meals dissolves uric acid. Pears are rich in pectin, calcium, phosphorus, potassium and vitamin A.

Linne (known also as Linnaeus), noted Swedish botanist, is said to have cured his gout with a diet of strawberries. The fruit is beneficial in the elimination of uric acid as well as other blood impurities. Fontenelle (1657-1757), noted French writer, attributed his long and active life to eating plenty of strawberries in season and preserves when fresh fruit was not available. Fontenelle apparently was not allergic to this luscious fruit.

Celery has been long esteemed in diet for people troubled with rheumatism or gout. A German recipe: For 2 months eat 2 cooked stalks of celery daily or drink the juice of the plant. A Japanese celery cure consists of celery cooked or raw in a variety of dishes to be taken for 1 month. The dishes exclude acid-forming ingredients, meats and foods containing oxalic acid such as spinach, rhubarb, sorrels, etc.

A letter from a California lady: "Now I want to give you a tried and true help for arthritis. My sister has it very bad and an old man told her to drink celery seed tea. She did and it has almost cured her. She drank 4 cups of the tea a day." The infusion is prepared like ordinary tea.

Consistent and free use of garden ripe tomatoes, eaten alone or in salads, juice or vegetable juice mixtures, helps elimination of uric acid as well as urea, one of the end products of metabolism excreted in the urine. Do not add salt. Tomatoes are not for sensitive people prone to allergies. *See Tomato in Part I.*

Raw or cooked apples eaten daily are very beneficial for gout or rheumatism. *Also see Apple Diet.*

In the early 1900s the Lemon Diet was in vogue. Dr. Fernie wrote: "The lemon treatment for making the blood aklaline against gouty acids in the system, is now gaining well-merited favor, unless carried to excess."

Lumbago: Instead of using your bundle of dill plant for pickles, try this old southern Europe and western Asia charm cure. Hang the dill over the door used most in your home. One probably needs a bit of faith-cure with this recipe.

Another: Wash the lumbar area with warm vinegar water. This should be done in a warm room.

A rustic recipe for pain in feet from rheumatism or gout: Rub painful parts with juice of onions.

A poultice of fresh grated root of horseradish is used as a counter-irritant for rheumatism, gout and sciatica. Horseradish is also used as a liniment by steeping the root in brandy or alcohol.

Red pepper (also called cayenne pepper, chilli or capsicum) is used in poultices and liniments for rheumatism, gout, arthritis, pleuritis, pericarditis and angina pectoris. The application in small doses stimultes a warm surface feeling, but left too long it can cause dermatitis and blistering.

SKIN

Strawberries have long been used by women in their relentless battle with wrinkles. The mashed fruit was rubbed into facial pores and allowed to remain on the face overnight, then washed off with clear water in the morning. The application also helps clean skin blemishes. The following is a simple and slightly astringent lotion: In a pint of white vinegar steep ½ pint of mashed strawberries. After several hours strain off the pulp and seeds. Enough rosewater may be added for fragrance.

The fresh juice of cucumbers is much used as a cosmetic to cleanse, lighten and soften the skin. Slices of cucumber may also be used instead of the juice. In either method the juice is allowed to dry on the skin. In Europe generally only the ripe yellow fruit is used. In U.S. the green unripe cucumber is used and probably is more astringent than the ripe fruit.

A handful of fresh chopped parsley greens steeped overnight is used in Europe to wash the face. It is said to leave the skin clean and smooth.

Summer freckles: Apply the juice of watercress, lemon juice, or the juice of parsley greens. In Germany people apply the water in which potatoes have been boiled for summer freckles as well as on frost-bites and it's said to be effective.

Sunburn: Apply honey.

Erysipelas: Apply honey to affected parts.

Skin rash: Apply fresh juice of black currant.

The pulverized dried seeds of kidney beans are dampened and applied to skin itch and rash. The seeds contain the alkaloid phaseoline.

An application of fresh sliced carrots relieves pruritis.

Raw onion rubbed on the skin also relieves itching.

Another: Rub inflamed part with lemon juice or sliced onion dipped in salt.

The inner leaves of fresh white cabbage, mashed to soften, are commonly used in European home practice as an application on pustules, skin rash, German measles, herpes and other skin troubles. *See Cabbage in Part I.*

SPRING CURE

Germans and Austrians call this "Frühlingskur or Frühjahrs-müdigkeit"—a deficiency condition caused by lack of vitamins from fresh fruits and vegetables lacking through winter months. Instead of dosing themselves with chemical vitamin pills, people sprinkle a variety of chopped fresh early spring greens on soups, stews, soft cheese, sauces, salads, broth, etc. Spring greens are particularly rich in vitamins. Among the most popular used are leeks, chives, cresses, dandelion and chervil.

Chervil is one of the most cherished plants in European gardens. Its lacy bright green leaves have a delicate and refreshing aroma that is especially appreciated on Frühlings-Suppe as well as on salads, sauces and salt boiled potatoes on which melted butter has been poured. Chervil should be fresh—not dehydrated. The minced herb is sprinkled on foods after cooking as heat destroys its fine aroma and delicate flavor. The plant is easily grown in temperate zones and is one of the earliest greens in spring.

Dandelion greens are one of the richest sources of vitamin A, containing 21,060 I.U. per cup compared to carrot which contains 15,220 I.U. per cup. This writer visited Bavaria and Austrian alpine regions in early spring and found valleys, meadows, waysides, gardens, and lawns abounding with the golden heads of this wonderful plant. André Voisin, member of The Academy of Agriculture in France, wrote, "In spring the flowers and stems of dandelion are enormously rich in estrogen." Dandelions, like other plants that flower very early in spring, obtain the materials necessary for the exhausting business of flower production from a store of food manufactured during the previous year. The dehydrated leaves of dandelion are brewed and used as a spring tonic. The root also has valuable medicinal uses for "lazy" livers. The roasted roots are used for making dandelion "coffee" which is almost indistinguishable from real coffee and possesses tonic and stimulant properties, yet lacks the possible injurious substance, caffeine.

From a book on old-fashioned beauty aids: "There is scarcely anything which can compare with spinach as a spring medicine and beautifier. The girl who religiously eats it as a Lenten diet, will blossom forth on Easter morning with a complexion that will rival the lilies by its fairness. Spinach contains salts of potassium, iron, and other things which conduce to long life and a fair skin, and is worth many bottles of cure for that tired feeling." *See Spinach and Dandelion in Part I.*

STOMACH

The author's aunt Mamie emphatically claimed there was nothing better for upset stomach than drinking a warm infusion of dried parsley greens made like ordinary tea.

One of grandmother's favorite foods for weak stomach or convalescence after stomach or colon operation was oatmeal porridge cooked with milk or water and sweetened with honey. Thin pea soup was also esteemed for weak stomach.

An authoritative German doctor wrote that ginger may be used for dyspeptic conditions of various types, but especially for subacid gastritis.

Warm ginger tea was popularly used by elderly folk as a stomach warmer.

The Family Herbal (1814) states: "Dyspeptic patients from hard drinking, and those subject to flatulency, have been known to receive considerable benefit by the use of Ginger tea; taking 2 or 3 cupfuls for breakfast, suiting it to their palate." Recipe for ginger tea: Pour 1 cupful of boiling water over a level tea-spoonful of dried Jamaica ginger. Drink when warm. Never boil ginger as heat dissipates its volatile (medicinal parts) oils. Saucer should be kept over cup in which ginger is steeping.

In small amounts, red pepper or chilli pepper stimulates the digestive juices. It should be avoided when there is inflammation.

Home remedy for dyspepsia, flatulence and vomiting: Take a small measure of paprika.

Sea-sickness: Take as much cayenne pepper or paprika as you can bear in a bowl of hot soup. It is said all nausea and squeamishness will disappear. Another: A cup of strong coffee, hot, without milk or sugar, is often successful.

In Germany cinnamon sticks steeped in red wine is popularly used in small doses for weak digestion of adults. Dr. J. Pereira stated that cinnamon in moderate doses stimulates the stomach, produces a sense of warmth in the epigastric region, and promotes the assimilative functions. Cinnamon tea checks nausea and vomiting.

Chewing a clove or two often relieves a nauseous feeling. A tea of cloves is said to tranquilize stomach cramps. The infusion should be taken in small doses.

Bilberry wine taken in small and regular doses is a popular European home remedy for digestive disturbances, weakness and loss of appetite. Bilberries (*Vaccinium myrtillus*) are very rich in provitamin A, vitamin C, mineral salts, glucoside, and organic acids.

Chewing a little horseradish root often relieves dyspepsia. The root must be fresh.

A half onion sliced thin and eaten with bread is a home remedy for flatulence and heartburn. Onions stimulate digestive juices, thus helping prevent putrid fermentation.

European peasants eat red currants or drink the juice for stomach discomfort caused by diet.

Heartburn: Thoroughly chew fresh carrots.

Nervous stomach: Drink a glass of warm milk with a dash of nutmeg or a few drops of the juice of garlic. The milk and nutmeg combination is also good for stomach cramps.

Rice well cooked in water is much used in diet in Germany for weak stomach.

Fully ripe bananas are easily digested and good for infants and older people with sensitive stomachs.

An old English source gives this recipe for debilitated stomach. Boil the juice of apples with equal quantity of sugar to make a syrup. Add a few tablespoonfuls of the syrup to a glass of cold water and drink frequently.

STOMACH ULCERS

Some years ago okra was given considerable publicity for its palliating effect for ulcer of the stomach. In a test with 17 patients a doctor reported 14 people treated with okra obtained immediate relief from their symptoms. One patient had no relief for 3 days after starting the okra treatment, but on the 5th day his symptoms disappeared. The tests were given with powdered okra which when combined with water makes a very rich mucilage. Taken internally it tends to neutralize acridity and forms a temporary protective coating over mucous membranes allowing inherent healing powers to restore normal functioning. The cut immature fresh pods in water also forms a thick mucilage. *See Okra in Part I.*

The Oxford Medical Adviser (Oxford University Press, 1931) states that junket is much used in the treatment of gastric ulcer and similar conditions. Junket consists of milk which has been acted upon by rennet. This forms a soft curd of the casein which is more easily digested than the curd which would naturally form in the stomach, and junket, therefore, forms a more easily digestible food than natural milk. If the curd is strained through muslin, whey is obtained which contains simply the water, sugar, and albuminous materials of the milk and is very easily digested.

Father Kneipp recommended a warm thick porridge of unrefined barley meal with milk to soothe stomach ulcers.

A porridge of oatmeal made with milk or water was also esteemed as a demulcent. To prepare oatmeal porridge stir 1 cup of oatmeal into 4 cups of water, allow to steep after stirring for a short time, bring to boiling point and steam for 3 hours.

The juice of white cabbage is used in the treatment of peptic and duodenal ulcers. The juice contains vitamin U, a factor that appears to be effective against peptic ulcer.

TENSION
On a trial with 900 students over a 3-year period a university research team found students who ate 2 apples a day had fewer tensions, headaches and emotional upsets than those who ate no apples.

Many French start off the day by drinking a glass of water in which a clove of crushed garlic has been steeped overnight.

An Austrian university professor and doctor wrote strawberries are cooling, calming and strengthening.

Tranquilizing: Drink slowly warm water well sweetened with honey—no side effects and no hangover—probably nothing else either for folk who live on stimulants trying to keep pace with modern machines.

In Europe the juice of common lettuce is still used as a mild sedative. The active principle is strongest when the plant goes to seed. George Fischer's *Heilkräuter und Arzneipflanzen* states, "er wirkt schwach beruhigend, opiumähnlich." Vinegar in lettuce salads neutralizes its soporific effects. Wild lettuce contains lactucarium and a scarce amount is present in cultivated species. Garden lettuce leaves (especially the outer leaves) are rich in iron and vitamins B_1, B_6, C and provitamin A.

WINTER FOODS

Meals high in sugars and starches or fats help offset the effect of cold weather on body temperature and the coordination of nerves and muscles. Rolled oats or the meal are good food for people who lead an active outdoor life.

Excellent winter dishes—*Soups:* onion soup with cheese, potato soup, soup with beans, peas, lentils. *Stews:* vegetables with meats, goulash with paprika. *Breakfast:* oatmeal, wheatgerm, bananas, dried fruits. *Beverages:* ginger tea, hot chocolate or milk.

WORMS

Tapeworms: Refrain from supper and breakfast on the following morning, and at 8 o'clock take ⅓ part of 200 minced pumpkin seeds, the shells of which have been removed by hot water; at 9 take another ⅓, at 10 the remainder, and follow it at 11 with strong dose of castor oil. Reputed to be the most harmless of all tapeworm recipes.—From *American Folk Medicine* by this author.

Peter Mertes' book *500 Heilpflanzen* (1936) claims the seeds of ripe cucumbers are effective against worms.

In European domestic practice a decoction made with water and the seeds of grapes or with wine and white cabbage seeds are used to expel worms.

Garlic cooked in milk or water is used in folk practice as an enema for maw-worms. Another source states: A clove of garlic when introduced into the lower bowel, will destroy thread worms, and, if eaten, will abolish round worms.

WOUNDS
A folk remedy for bad healing wounds or festering ulcers was an application of garlic juice or the juice mixed with pure honey. The wad of cotton wool used to apply the medicine should be burned—not used a second time.

In World War I the English used the expressed juice of garlic with a little distilled water on sphagnum moss as an application to wounds for prevention of suppuration or sepsis.

Festering ulcers: Apply a thick slice of fried onion and renew the application several times with fresh fried slices. Another German physician wrote that raw onions may be used as an application.

A salve made with finely minced onions mixed with honey and a little vinegar is commonly used in domestic practice for minor open wounds. *See Onion and Garlic in Part I.*

A recipe from a household medical guide written by a doctor in the days when doctors, hospitals, clinics, specialists, etc. were scarce or non-existent: For wounds made by rusty tools and nails, bruises, and lacerated wounds, take raw salt pork and about the same bulk in boiled onions, chop together thoroughly fine in a wooden bowl and apply warm. Bind on about ½-inch thick on the injured or wounded parts.

German recipe for gangrenous wounds: Apply thoroughly cleaned slices or minced carrot roots to the part and renew the application with fresh roots every hour.

A poultice for ulcers: Heat grated raw potatoes and apply as hot as can be tolerated. Johann Künzle, noted Swiss herbalist, advised applying slices of raw potato on gangrenous wounds. Künzle added that wounds heal faster when one avoids meats and sour foods.

Ulcers and slow healing wounds: Thoroughly wash and dry several inner leaves of white cabbage and remove their larger veins. Wash and soften the leaves with the round end of a clean bottle; lay the mashed leaves over the wound and bandage. Repeat application morning and night with fresh leaves. It is important that the application is perfectly clean. Cabbage leaves were used since ancient times for wounds.

A rustic recipe for gangrenous wounds: Make a poultice of clean mashed rotten apples. Another source mentions the juice pressed from rotten apples is used on a poultice. The poultice should be body-warm and renewed frequently with new bandage as well as juice. Both recipes are from sources on folk medicine. The author found no other mention regarding rotten apples. It is possible that apples in this state are rich in enzymes and may have antibacterial action. This recipe should not be tested by a layman as it may be dangerous, especially if the apples have been sprayed with toxic chemicals. *See Apples in Part I.*

European rustics apply pure honey to open or festering small wounds. The fresh juice of ripe (yellow) cucumbers is also used for wounds and bedsores.

In World War II German soldiers carried dehydrated lemon pectin in their emergency kits to be used on wounds in order to form a clot quickly.

An English physician wrote that rice flour dusted on a bleeding wound or sore will effectually stop the flux.

A poultice made of unrefined barley meal was used on ulcers and abcesses in old-time practice. German sources say this application is "vorzüglich" (superior).

The pulverized dried and shelled seeds of pumpkin are used in home practice as a healing agent on wounds.

Bibliography

Anshutz, E. P. *New and Old Forgotten Remedies.* 1900.

Ashley, R. and Duggal, H. *Dictionary of Nutrition.* 1976.

Ayer, H. H. *Harriet Hubbard Ayer's Book of Health and Beauty.* 1902.

Bardeau, Fabrice. *Die Apotheke Gottes.* 1978.

Blüchel, Kurt. *Heilkräfte der Natur.* 1977.

Böhme, Dr. Carl. *Was muss man von den Heilpflanzen wissen?* 1904.

Boros, Dr. Georges. *Unsere Heil- und Teepflanzen: 1.* 1963.

———. *Unsere Heil- und Teepflanzen: 2.* 1965.

Braun, Dr. Hans. *Heilpflanzen Lexikon.* 1971.

Comrie, John D. *Oxford Medical Advisor for the Home.* 1931.

Dyk, Anton, M.D. and Leo, Proksch. *Gesund durch Heiltees und Heilkräuter.* 1972.

Fernie, W. T., M.D. *Meals Medicinal.* 1905.

Fischer, Eugen. *Heil Pflanzen.* 1951.

Fischer, Georg. *Heilkräuter und Arzneipflanzen.* 1966.

Fischer, Dr. Wilhelm J. *Heilpflanzen der Heimat.* 1937.

Flach, Grete. *Aus Meinem Rezept-Schatzkästlein.* 1977.

Freidenwald, J., M.D. and Ruhrah, J., M.D. *Diet in Health and Disease.* 1925.

Gäbler, Hartwig. *Das Büchlein von den heilenden Kräutern.* n.d.

Göök, Roland. *Gewürze und Kräuter von A–Z.* n.d.

Gudden, Barbara. *Heilende Kräuter.* n.d.

Hertwig, Hugo. *Knaurs Heilpflanzen Buch.* 1954.

Hlava, Bohumir and Lanska, Dagmar. *Lexikon der Küchen und Gewurzkräuter.* 1977.

Köbl, Conrad. *Kräuterfibel.* 1972.

Künzle, Johann. *Gesunder Körper durch Heilkräuter.* n.d.

Lassel, M. *Gesundheit und Kraft durch Kräutergold.* 1954.

Masefield, G. B., Wallis, M., Harrison, S. G., and Nicholson, B. E. *The Oxford Book of Food Plants.* 1969.

Merle, Gibbons and Reitch, John, M.D. *The Domestic Dictionary.* 1842.

Mertes, Peter. *500 Heilpflanzen.* 1936.

Meyer, Clarence. *American Folk Medicine.* 1973.
──── . *Herbal Recipes.* 1978.
Meyer, Joseph E. *The Herbalist.* 1918.
Nelson, Alexander. *Medical Botany.* 1951.
Nielsen, Harald and Hancke, Verner. *Heilpflanzen in Farbe.* 1976.
──── . *Giftpflanzen.* 1979.
Pahlow, Mannfried. *Heilpflanzen heute.* n.d.
──── . *Heilpflanzen Kompass.* n.d.
Polunin, Oleg. *Flowers of Europe.* 1969.
Quinche, Robert and Bossard, Eugen. *Gewürzkräuter.* 1976.
Ritter, Dr. T. J. *Mother's Remedies.* 1922.
Rogler, August. *Kräutersegen.* n.d.
Rogler, Gustl. *Kräuterwunder.* 1949.
Rüdt, Ulrich. *Heil- und Giftpflanzen.* 1973.
Schauenberg, Paul and Paris, Ferdinand. *BLV Bestimmungsbuch Heilpflanzen.* 1969.
Schönfelder, Bruno and Fischer, Wilhelm. *Welche Heilpflanzen Ist Das?* 1968.
Simonis, Werner-Christian. *Taschenbuch der Heil und Gewürzkräuter.* 1957.
Stary, Fr. and Jirasek, V. *Heilpflanzen kennen, sammeln, anwenden.* 1972.
Trauter, Eva. *Das Heyne Gewürzbuch.* 1966.
Wallnöfer, Dr. Heinrich. *Gesund durch Gewürze.* 1968.
Willfort, Richard. *Gesundheit durch Heilkräuter.* 1971.

Index